Yesterday in Haiti

The Journals of a Missionary Nurse

Pat Bramhall

WestBow
PRESS
A DIVISION OF THOMAS NELSON

WestBow Press books may be ordered through booksellers or by contacting:

WestBow Press
A Division of Thomas Nelson
1663 Liberty Drive
Bloomington, IN 47403
www.westbowpress.com
1-(866) 928-1240

ISBN: 978-1-4497-1371-3 (sc)
ISBN: 978-1-4497-1373-7 (dj)
ISBN: 978-1-4497-1372-0 (e)

Library of Congress Control Number: 2011924135

Printed in the United States of America

WestBow Press rev. date: 5/13/2011

Lovingly dedicated to
Kathy and Alice

Many special thanks to Mike Vassar for helping this computer illiterate with all the technicalities involved with this project. I could never have done it without his help.

Getting There

"After you have corrected me, I will thank you by living as I should. I will obey!"

Psalm 119:7&8 LB

"No, dear brothers, I am still not all I should be, but I am bringing all my energies to bear on this one thing: Forgetting the past, and looking forward to what lies ahead, I strain to reach the end of the race and receive the prize for which God is calling us up to Heaven, because of what Christ Jesus did for us."

Phil. 3:13&14 LB

December, 1984   In California

This journal has been lying in my dresser drawer for a year now, and when I first got it, it was with the idea of writing down "My Life's Adventures" (really MIS-adventures), but tonight they seem to have paled in the light of the Light of the World. I can see that they are not, and never have been, anything worth writing about. Rather, things and a life to be ashamed of, rather than to be written about.

Since August of 1983 when I left Northern California, and came to live here in Southern California with my mother, I have had a whole new life open up. It's been a year of surprises – wonderful things that the Savior has done for me.

It started with my plan of going back to Saudi Arabia. I was, I thought, looking for God's will. I found a tape of John MacArthur's titled, "God's Will Is Not Lost". It sounded interesting, so I listened to it on my way to work one day. It surely WAS interesting, and it really hit me, and spoke to my heart. He said, "If you want to know God's will, you first have to know God." He spoke about obedience and purity in a Christian's life, and I decided for once to really BE obedient.

I began to clean up the dark corners of my life, really seeing for the first time how I had been deceiving myself. I thought I had been a Christian for over forty years, but I had never been willing to be obedient. Instead, I was like Adam, and blamed God for my sin, by saying, "Well, God, YOU made me like this." I really saw this for the first time, for what it was, and for the first time, admitted it for what it was – MY sin.

I will confess to you now, what sin that was. I had to tell the elders at Grace Church, that I had been married and divorced four times. I hated to have to do it, but I knew I had to be completely honest with them. I knew that the Lord had forgiven me, but I found it was more difficult to have your fellow man forgive you, or to forget the past, as God is willing to do.

How gracious and how merciful the Lord has been; how patient and long suffering toward me. He should have abandoned me, or slain me, but instead, He was always there, waiting, right beside me. I have tried to get away from Him; I have 'tuned out', and quenched the Holy Spirit. His 'temple' has been a place I'm sure He has been very unhappy in, but He never left it. I have grieved Him over and over, but still He stayed – wooing and comforting me when I turned to Him in my own sin caused grief. I have been like the wicked, selfish Children of Israel, and like them, I have been wandering in my own self-made wilderness! Forty years lost, that can never be retrieved.

Only God can make something of the years He chooses to leave to me, and those years will be wholly His! For whatever He may choose to do with my life, it is His. I want only His will, as I have discovered the joy unspeakable that comes only with communion that is unbroken by sin. As Jim Elliott, the young man martyred by the Auca Indians in 1955, wrote in his journal, that God would ". . .light these idle sticks of my life, that I might burn up for Thee." So I pray that even though the sticks of my life are much shorter now, so much having been consumed by my own selfishness, I pray that He will light BOTH ends, and let me burn out for Him, for His glory.

I was reading in II Timothy 2:20-21, about different dishes in a home, being made for different uses. What a practical thing, that a woman understands. It speaks of some dishes that are made of gold, and some of silver to be used on special occasions, and for guests. They are things of beauty, and are made to bring praise to the one who owns them. Then, it speaks of dishes made of wood, and some made of clay. They are not expensive, and are used for the kitchen, and to put the garbage in. They are for the menial, 'every day living' uses.

I know that my opportunity to be a vessel of gold or silver for special uses is gone. I threw it away when I chose a life of disobedience, but, *"Oh, my Gracious Master, just let me be a vessel of wood or clay – at least to be useful and usable for even the most menial of tasks – gathering up what's left after the meal; it doesn't matter, Lord. I don't ask for any fancy task, or one to be seen by men – just to be usable."*

The Lord has shown me so many things that I already knew, but I had never applied them to my life. *"Make me now, an obedient 'doer' of the Word."* What a joy!

He is loosing, finger by finger, my grasp on the things of this world. I am reduced to one room in my mother's house; I have been trying for twenty years to make a 'nest' for myself –now, it really isn't important anymore. I have a home in Heaven now, where my Savior sits enthroned, and I am learning, by the presence of the Holy Spirit, to live in the Heavenlys! All the things that I was hanging onto have been slowly slipping from my fingers, and oh, the JOY that He has given in their place! The things that were so important a year ago are becoming less and less important. Oh, for God given priorities!

"Take me Lord, to the place where nothing on this earth holds me to it, but where loosing my grip, I am not empty – but conversely – filled by the things that only You can give. Teach me to abide in the Vine, to be a branch that will bear much fruit for Thy glory."

I am going to try to write in this book throughout the new year of 1985, which will soon be upon us. I doubt that I will write anything in here that will be very profound, or that will impress anyone, but I pray, something that will bring glory to my Lord, and perhaps comfort or encourage another who might someday take the time to read it.

I thank God for the teaching ministry of John MacArthur, and for Grace Community Church. I joined the church in the summer and it's the first time I am proud – poor choice of words – to be a part of a church family. I really feel like a part of a body, and the Lord has given me a ministry there in the tape library, that I love. I mentioned how my walk back to the Lord was begun by the Spirit through one of John MacArthur's tapes. Well, now I'm working in the tape library at Grace Community Church on Sunday mornings, and it thrills my heart to be able to put into so many hands tapes that I know the Spirit will bless and use to bring honor to the Lord, and joy to the hearers when they apply the Truth that they hear to their own lives. I have listened to tape after tape, and each one has brought me closer and closer to Him.

I thank God every day for John. He is so faithful in teaching the Word, and glorifying Christ. He only teaches the Word, verse by verse, using the Old Testament for illustration, and never giving his opinion, only giving the Word alone, and showing you how to apply it to your own life in obedience. I love it, and I thank God for giving me a part in getting the Word out. I have even been able to share some tapes with some at work.

God has promised that His Word will never return to Him void, but will accomplish the purpose for which it was sent out. I have a great hunger for the Word now, and I could read it and listen to it being expounded all day long.

"Thank you Savior, for your blessed Word; I long to know it better, as it is the power of God in our dealings with others. It is the power that leads us to salvation, and I want to be a workman that has it flowing out of my heart and my mouth that others may come to know Him, whom to know aright is Life Eternal."

John read a wonderful poem on one of his tapes one day, and I want to write it in here now. I feel it describes me – a bird with a broken wing.

"Like a bird that trails a broken wing, I have come home to Thee.
Home from a flight and freedom, that was never meant for me.
And I, who have known far spaces, and the fierce heat of the sun,
Ask only the shelter of Thy wings, now that the day is done.

I have written a second verse, because I don't believe that God wants us to just hide forever under His wing. There is work to be done, so here is my verse:

"Oh, Thou who hast created me, mend my broken wing,
And send me upward again in flight, and give me Thy song to sing.
A song of joy to glorify Thee, with every beat of my wing,
Until in Heaven, I see Thy face, and a new song I will sing!"

"Keep me Lord, from flying where I should not, and thus I will avoid meeting the Prince of the Power of the Air – the Hawk, who would kill me with his cruel talons of hate, rending my wings, to send me falling, crippled to the Earth – useless for the task to which You have sent me in flight. Energize my wings by the Power of Thy Spirit, that my flight will be swift and sure!" (I'm not used to flying, Lord.)

December 11, 1984

I have been thinking about Prairie Bible Institute, in Three Hills, Alberta, Canada. Maybe going back, and taking all the classes to prepare myself for some type of ministry. I want only what my Master wants for my life, as it is wholly His. I don't want to jump ahead, or make a mistake. I pray that He will teach me to follow, as He has already promised to lead us. We don't have to ask to be led, He has already said He would do that, but we do need to ask Him to teach us to follow. He is the Good Shepherd, and I am one sheep He has had to rescue too often. I want to follow Him so closely now, that when His foot is lifted, mine will come down into the print His has just made. I won't be able to see beyond His back, but praise God, I don't have to see, I only have to follow! He has traveled the path before, and I will trust Him.

December 13, 1984

I worked last night, and initially wanted to work with Maggie to be able perhaps to speak more with her about the Savior. Instead, she was in charge and sent me to the Preemie room to work with Maria. How absolutely marvelous to be quiet, and know that He – the sovereign God-knows, and has a plan for each of us, every day. I really hadn't thought much about Maria, it was Maggie I was concerned for, but God was after Maria! I was able to speak much with her about the sufficiency of Jesus Christ, and all that He has done for us. She was very receptive, and I believe she is an honest, seeking soul. The Holy Spirit had prepared her heart wonderfully, and I pray that tonight she may tell me that she has accepted Jesus as her Savior and Lord. God is surely able – praise His wonderful Name! What peace to rest in Him in all things!

December 17, 1984

My mother and I arrived home tonight after driving all the way from Tonopah, Nevada, where my two sons live. We spent a day and two nights with my son Jim and his three little girls. His wife, Pam, had gone to Reno.

I had driven all day Saturday, and just arrived in Tonopah, when it began to snow. It snowed all night, and Sunday morning was beautiful.

Jim gave a good Sunday School lesson in Isaiah on true worship. I am so blessed by, and so proud of my two sons. Praise God, they know and love the Lord, and are living for Him. I pray God will use them mightily in that Tonopah mission field.

Sunday night we went to a community program put on by all of the different churches in Tonopah. Jeff and Jim didn't sing in the choir as they were uncertain as to whether that should, since it was composed of Catholic, Mormon, Pentecostal, Lutheran, Baptist, etc. They felt that since there were those whose teachings were scripturally unsound, that they shouldn't participate. I said that I felt that as long as the program was glorifying to the Lord, maybe it was OK. Then Jim asked, " Would it have been OK for the Children of Israel to call in some of the Philistines to help them sing?" Good question!

It was very cold Sunday night, and walking around in the crunching snow brought back memories of Christmases at Prairie Bible Institute in Canada. I am feeling very moved to go there in April for the graduation, to be at the Lord's disposal, and to be exposed to all of it again, and see what the Lord will show me.

The ride home today was spectacular, as far as the scenery went. Beautiful rugged mountains, white with snow, with a long ribbon of clouds decorating the sloping sides. Along the sides of the road, the sagebrush and grass were encased in ice. The sun was just at an angle to shine through the ice, and on it, to create thousands of brilliantly decorated 'Christmas trees', gleaming, and reflecting the light. It was so beautiful! It's hard to imagine that it will all be even more beautiful, when the curse is lifted from it, than what is was today. And how easy it was for God to decorate His creation as we could never have done, and He did it overnight! Miles and miles of gleaming beauty, just in a moment. Praise His Name!

We brought Jim's little girl Tina with us, and she was just singing about Jesus in her tiny little voice from the back seat. How precious is this little two and a half year old girl.

December 18, 1984

"For I, the Lord thy God, will hold thy right hand, saying unto thee, "Fear not; I will help thee."

Isaiah 41:13 KJV

I found this verse on a card the other day, and it was so true to what I was trying to say concerning my own testimony. How, even though I wandered away, He never let me go completely, for His hand was holding on to mine, always gently drawing me back to His side. During the insecure moments of my life, when I feel unprotected and defenseless, I fear I will loosen my grip on my Heavenly Father's hand. As a flash of panic sets in, and my soul grows disquieted within, I hear my Father's voice speak His soothing words of comfort, "Don't be anxious about how firm the grip of your hand is on mine. . . . for my hand is holding on to yours, and nothing will cause it to slacken. Even in your most troubled hour, I will not allow you to pull away."

He didn't, Praise God!

January 20, 1985

We had a great guest speaker at Grace today, Ron Stedman from Palo Alto. He spoke on Romans 12:1-3, and during his message, he mentioned God holding onto our hands, and Jubilant Sykes also sang a song about God holding onto our hands.

Again, the idea of our safe keeping is not dependent on how tightly we can cling to His hand, but rather on the fact that He is holding on to our hand. He will never let go of our hand or let us fall all the way down, or allow another to tear our hand away from His. Instead, He will never let go of us no matter how weak we are, nor how loose our grip upon His hand is – He holds on to our hand forever! Halleluiah!

Saw a film on the Moslem world tonight, and heard there are more missionaries in Alaska than in the entire Moslem world. I can understand this, having lived in Saudi Arabia for two years. The Moslem people have to be one of the most, if not THE most, difficult people in the world to evangelize. For one thing, there are so few men to go to them, and they would never speak to a woman. They are so brainwashed about their religion, and are so afraid to go against their leaders to even listen. No one is allowed to speak to a Moslem about Jesus Christ, even though they consider Him to be a prophet. When I was in Saudi Arabia, one sure way to be deported was to talk to a Moslem person about Christ. I believe that Islam is indeed Satan's own counterfeit, in direct opposition to true Christianity.

"Make me faithful Lord, here, over the small things, or I'll never know anything more."

January 27, 1985

"Oh, Lord, You alone are my hope; I've trusted you since childhood."

Psalm 71:5 LB

"And, now, in my old age, don't set me aside. Don't forsake me now when my strength is failing."

Psalm 71:9 LB

I don't know how old David was when he says he "has trusted God from childhood," but I was ten years old when I read about the very thing John preached on today: the illegal, unjust trial, and murder of Jesus. When they had finally gotten Jesus to say He was God, they were triumphant in that now they could kill Him for blasphemy. They pronounced their sentence, and then – they spit on Him! Jesus was executed not for saying He was God, but for being the God He said He was! They called it blasphemy that He said He was God, but they, themselves were the blasphemers!

I realized, even as a child, that He had taken my place there, and that I was the guilty one, as guilty as those who spat upon Him, the beautiful loving Savior, whose only acts were those of tenderness, kindness, and love. Then they hit Him, blindfolded Him and mocked Him. He could have called 10,000 angels to destroy those men, and set Him free, but instead He was silent – for you, and for me. Shall I not fill my mouth with praise for Him?

Then, in verse 9 of Psalm 71 – How I pray that God will not "set me aside in my old age," but instead will make me as verse 14 in Psalm 92 says, "Even in old age they will produce fruit, and be vital and green." Then, verse 15 gives my reason for desiring this – "This honors the Lord, and exhibits His faithful care. . ."

How faithful He has been to me – Oh, that I may bear fruit to honor Him.

"Let me burn out Lord, for Thee, consume my life, engulf it in the flame of Your Spirit! It may not burn for very long, but may it be bright enough to give light to some who now sit in darkness. And how dark is that darkness!"

February 3, 1985

Another wonderful Sunday spent at the Savior's feet. I wish the weeks were 6 days of Sundays, and one day to work! Both messages were very good today, and the music is soul lifting, and SO beautiful!

I thank God for another chance, every day I go to work, to speak to someone about the Lord. Yet, when I am speaking, I sometimes think about how this must sound to them. I hear myself as they must hear me, and I can't help but think how foolish it might sound to them. I feel so inept in speaking for the Savior. The things that are so real in my life and heart, I know must seem ridiculous to them. Is it that I am afraid of seeming foolish to them? What a trap that is to fall into. The fear of man! When He has told us to not be afraid of their faces!

How much easier, I think sometimes, it would be to die for Christ, than it is to live for Him. We are so frail, and so easily tripped up. Yet, His word promises that He will catch us, and enable us, and I know that there have been times when I have wondered as I spoke, *"Where did THAT come from?"* Those were the times when I knew it was the Lord speaking.

"Oh, that my vision and my thoughts would be tuned only to Him that I might be filled to overflowing, and not 'trying' in the flesh, but simply being so filled with Him that He will overflow onto those around me without my 'trying', or even knowing. Then it will be all of Him, and none of me." That is what a vessel is for.

Oh, to be just a suit of working clothes the Spirit would wear today! I feel very good, and at peace about going to Prairie in April. I even have my vacation time on the schedule at work – Praise the Lord! I feel so sure there will be answers to the seeking for direction for my life there. I really do want some kind of full time service, but it may be that this is not His will for me. I feel I must take this step for now.

February 10, 1985

Yesterday was my little grand-daughter Heather's birthday. (How soon they are no longer babies, and how soon accountable.) I Praise the Lord, with thanksgiving, for answered prayer in my little grand-son Jeffrey's asking Jesus to come into his heart! I have been praying that these precious little grand-children would early come to know the One, who will stick by them, give meaning, joy, and fullness to their lives that the world will promise, but can never give. Outside of Christ there is no meaning or joy to life. In fact, there is NO LIFE outside of Christ.

We had a beautiful baptism service tonight. I really enjoy the testimonies people give, and each is so unique in the way God has brought each person to Himself. One tiny Philippine lady, with tears streaming down her face, very movingly (it brought tears running down my face) told of her lonely quest, searching for the meaning of life. She had been raised in a Catholic home, and in her longing for God, she had gone into a convent. God, she said, brought her out, and she went to school, thinking education would satisfy the longing. She tried many religions, and some cults, always with the same results – no change, and no peace. For awhile, she became depressed, then she became angry and negative toward everyone, and everything – even against God. Finally, in desperation, she went to her knees, and cried out to God, " Oh, God, if You are there, show Yourself to me! Come into my life, and give me peace. I am so small in Your sight, and so unworthy, but I ask for Your forgiveness and Your presence."

And then, she said, for the first time in her life, she felt her burden lifted, and great peace came over her whole being. What a beautiful testimony, and so simply and humbly given.

I admire everyone who stands there in the water, and speaks out for the Lord, telling three thousand people how they came to know Him. It can't be easy. But then, our God doesn't call us to the easy things, does He? I have wondered if I could do it. I have difficulty speaking to one or two, but to three thousand!

I have gotten a preliminary questionnaire from Wycliffe Bible Translators. I will fill it out, and send it to them, trusting the Lord to tell them that I am truly His now, and I am in His will. I hate to have to tell them about my 'soap opera' past, but I know I must be honest and open, so God will be able to lead me. I doubt that my nursing experience will be what they need, but the Lord knows. I also ran across – in the book I am reading, "Shadow of the Almighty" – a mention of the Bible Institute of Los Angeles' Medical School, which I had forgotten about. Maybe I'll see what they have to offer. I am really looking forward to going to Prairie in April, Lord willing. I'm hoping for some answers from the Lord there. What peace to know that He goes before me, and His footprints are there for me to follow.

The Good Shepherd never pushes His sheep from behind, or lets them wander, not knowing the way. He always goes before them; He knows the right path and He leads them. He has promised to lead us – we don't have to keep asking for guidance, only for help in following! He is the Shepherd we can surely trust, because we know He loves His sheep, for He gave His life for them.

I feel like a sheep. I've been feeding in the green pasture of Grace Church, feasting, and getting very fat. I would love to just stay here and get fatter and fatter on the rich spiritual food we get here every Sunday. But, I know the only reason for fattening sheep, is to slaughter them, to feed others. *"Oh, Father, You know when that will be, and I am Your sheep, to do with as You will. May I be willing to go from the feasting, into Your courts with praise, to be a sacrifice that others may live."*

I sat next to a Japanese girl tonight, and noticed she was reading a Japanese Bible. How does one underline a verse when it is read vertically instead of horizontally?

John told about his trip to Chicago last week, and a thought came to me. I have been praying that God would send someone to tell my lost son Tommy, about the Lord, that he too might know the joy of knowing Christ. I gave him to the Lord, privately when he was born, and publicly when he was three years old, and today I thought, maybe he has heard John speak there in Chicago. He is on the radio there, and it is not an impossibility. Not with my God!

February 11, 1985

What a God we have! He is the God of miracles, and the unexpected. I got up this morning and decided to take my car and get the brakes fixed. I took along my tape player and my embroidery to occupy myself while I waited. As I was sitting there embroidering tiny chicks on my granddaughter's dress and listening to John, someone came in, and sat down next to me. As I looked up, I couldn't believe my eyes – it was the same little Philippine lady that had been baptized last night, and that I had just written about. The very one that I had been so blessed by as I had listened to her testimony! I took off my earphones, and said, "What's your name?" I remembered the lady had said last night that her name was Cora. She looked at me a bit startled, and said, "Cora."

I then told her that I had watched her baptism last night, and told her how her testimony had really blessed and encouraged me. We began to talk about it, and for the next two hours I listened, spellbound, as she told me more of what the Lord had done in her life. One miracle after another, she was moved along by God. He has provided everything she has needed, from transportation – and I don't mean just a car for here to there – I mean a plane ride from Denmark to the United States, protection from one she was afraid was going to kill her, places to live in countries where she knew no one, and couldn't speak the language – it was just awesome. How wonderful to hear someone who has experienced these kinds of things, and how encouraging to be reminded again of what a truly remarkable God we serve.

She told me of how she went to Moody Bible Institute, because she wanted to learn the Bible. She arrived at O'Hare airport, alone, not knowing her way around at all. Someone had given her directions to the school, so she followed the directions given, and got on a bus. After she had gotten on, and was on the way, she discovered it was not the right bus. She told someone that she was on the wrong bus, that she wanted to go to Moody Bible Institute. They told her that the directions she had been given were wrong, and she was on the right bus! This is just an example of so many wonderful things she told me. What a treat, and blessing for me! What a great day! I could never have planned it, but God did.

March 17, 1985

I just haven't had the heart to write in this, even though the flow goes on. A few more Sundays to have the privilege of being a part of Grace Church, and the many ministries there, have gone by.

About ten days ago I received an answer to my preliminary questionnaire to Wycliffe. It was a very sensitive and really nice letter, and one that I'm sure was very difficult for someone to have to write. They said that in view of what I had written, they would not be able to use me. It was a big disappointment, but I know it was from the Lord. I have this written in my Bible – 'Disappointment is His appointment'

I guess I haven't honestly faced the possibility that, perhaps God won't be able to use me in the way that I desire. I've always been able to work things around to the way I wanted them, but no more. Now, I only want what He wants, His will, not mine. It may very well be just what I don't really want, which is – to stay here. I keep saying that I will be satisfied if I know that it is His will, but it is a struggle to quietly hope, and wait.

And yet, after such flagrant disobedience, how can I expect Him to use me as He might have if I had only learned these lessons earlier, and been obedient to what I knew was right.

If Moses was denied entry into the Promised Land because of his sin, and if a whole generation of people died in the desert, and weren't allowed to go in, who am I, that I should expect to go unpunished? Forgiveness? Yes! Praise God, yes. I am His, and I am forgiven, and, yes, Heaven is mine, because of the sacrifice of Christ, but I may not be given the joy of such service for Him here. It breaks my heart, but then I think of how I broke His loving heart with my sinful life. How I wish that I had had the teaching early in my life that I have had here. It might have made a difference.

I look at the beautiful young people here, with their lives before them, and I envy them the opportunity that is theirs for years of service, and perhaps a Christian partner, and I can't help but wish that it had happened to me, before I made such wrong choices in my desire to have my own way.

I wonder about going to Prairie for the conference. Whether it's really the thing to do, and yet for some reason, I just feel that I must go. I'm sometimes tempted to just say – Forget it! – and take a nice trip instead, but I can not. I will obey! More and more, I am convicted of my poor stewardship of my time and my money. I'm going to get a refund of four thousand dollars from the government, and the state. And I thought I'd have to pay! Isn't God good! I wish I were brave enough to give it all away, but I'm not really sure that would be His will either. I don't feel free to just spend it, so I'll wait on His directive.

I was hoping my friend Lisa, would go to Prairie with me, but she feels she can't, so I'll go alone. Always alone, yet never alone. Perhaps my broken wing will never be flight worthy again. Even if I'm grounded, my feet still work, and I can walk. Earth bound – but only for a time, thank god!

April 14, 1985

Tomorrow I leave for Prairie, and I really don't know why. I am going, believing that God has something for me there – some directive for my life. I pray the Holy Spirit will make me sensitive, and keep my eyes, ears, and heart open to Him. I'm hoping to be able to talk to some representatives of mission boards, to see if I can fit in somewhere.

I went to a missionary candidate meeting at Grace, and Mr. Wong, an elder there, said he would follow up on my question of mission needs for nurses. He doesn't know about my past, however. I fear it may prove to be the millstone around my neck. And yet, I'm forgiven, am I not? By Christ, but not by men? I can see their side of the question; they need those who've proven faithful, and trustworthy, and I surely have not done so in my past. Does that mean I will never be trusted again?

I've even begun to wonder whether I was really saved so long ago. John has shaken me somewhat, and I almost wish I could say, no, I was not. Then I could not be held accountable for my past, but I'm just not sure. Sounds like an easy way out, but could I really have lived as I did, and been a Christian? I surely feel different about obedience now than I did then. Then I blamed God, saying it wasn't my fault because He had made me the way I was – with a hunger that couldn't be satisfied.

I have been asking myself, what is my real motive for wanting to go to the mission field? I have to admit, I wouldn't be going to be a preacher to preach Christ, but rather to be an example of Christ, and give my life to these people. I want to serve, not some strange people, necessarily, but to serve Christ in the most giving way I can. I want to give every thing I am and have, in real physical service to Him. I think of Mary Slessor who gave of herself everyday for others in Africa; who had no comforts or ease, not even necessities like sleep. I think of Mother Theresa, who is an example of what a Christian should be doing, in giving her life in service, not as works to win Salvation, but as service to the Master we love.

I love the Lord, and I long to give my life away for Him, that when I stand before Him, I will not be ashamed. I want Him to be pleased with me, and with my life, but right now, even I am not pleased with it. I want to serve others in need, because the only way I know to serve Christ is by serving others.

The Biblical definition of love is, "self sacrificing service to others."

"In as much as ye have done it unto the least of these my brethren, ye have done it unto me," Jesus said.

I am not meant to preach. I am not gifted as a teacher, but I know how to care for the hurting bodies of those who suffer, especially the little bodies. I know there are small ones somewhere who need that care. I wouldn't be missed from the work force here, and there, I would probably BE the work force.

"Oh, Lord, mend my broken wing, and let me fly – for Thee! I know I am asking for more than I deserve, but He has said "to ask."

April 16, 1985   Prairie Bible Institute

I arrived in Three Hills, Alberta, Canada around noon after a pleasant drive from Calgary. Rented a motel room for a night, and went and changed my clothes. (I felt uncomfortable at Prairie in slacks.)

I roamed for awhile in their book room, noting several of John's books, and one tape. Then I went into town and walked up and down the main street – that took about five minutes. I saw the big old house we lived in for the first three years Andy and I went to school here, and visited the places where our children had played. Then, I went back to the school to register for the conference.

I went out and walked around the campus, trying to remember the years when we were here. Some very happy memories; they reminded me that it was a good start, but went bad because of me.

I remembered the Tabernacle, which is their main auditorium, but when I went inside, it was in a rather sorry state. I was amazed at the size of it. It's only about half the size of Grace Church, and yet when we were here, I remember how huge it seemed to us.

Lots of memories of a happier time came rushing back when I walked over to the married couples housing, called the 'motels', where we had lived for Andy's last year. I saw a group of kids playing, just like my kids played there, and a group of young men sitting outside discussing who knows what – maybe where they will go after graduation. I pray they won't end up like Andy and I did – on the shelf.

I look at all these bright beautiful young people, with their lives before them, ready and equipped to go out for the Lord, and I wonder how I could have made such a terrible mistake. I also wonder how I could have gone all those years listening to Mr. Maxwell, and then so willfully decide to be so disobedient because I couldn't have my own way. Was I really saved? I couldn't pray with anyone, and Andy and I never prayed together. I was always unhappy, and wanting what I couldn't have. I hid it well, and I knew the right words to say, but inside, I knew I was not being honest. It wasn't really me, and inside I knew I was wrong.

Tears kept coming to my eyes everywhere I went, and I felt that people were looking at me in a strange way. I really felt like a misfit – and I was always alone. I even sat and ate alone. No one ever sat down at the table with me. I felt like a moral leper. Here I am, I love the Lord, I want to serve Him, but my past is clinging to me. *Where do I go from here, dear Lord, where do I go to get around this high wall I am facing? Oh, how bitter is the bitterness of regret! I wonder if Moses cried when he learned he wouldn't be allowed to go into the Promised Land?*

Prairies divorce policy – you can go to school, but you can't graduate.

April 18, 1985

This experience is somewhat similar to a roller-coaster ride, up, and then down! Wonderful message last night by Elisabeth Elliott. Now, there is a lady who really has it all together. Sure wish I could sit down and open my heart to her, as I really need some words of advice. She is a no nonsense person, and I'm a little bit afraid of what she would tell me.

I'm finding it difficult to enjoy the mission's seminar, because I want to do everything I see. I saw a good film on Missionary Aviation Fellowship. What a wonderful ministry; I'd love to be in that helicopter going out into the jungle to save that "poor dying baby" but I'm afraid that's not for me. It's hard to know that you could help, and be useful, but because of a stupid mistake in the past, it's out of reach.

Today, I've been feeling like I must have a big 'D' burned on my forehead. I don't think Prairie would let me in as a student, certainly not to be on staff as a nurse.

I'm afraid I am feeling a root of bitterness here that must go! I know a tiny bit of how David must have felt. He's another example of sin forgiven, but not without the penalty, or the 'rod of correction'. He was not allowed to build the Temple he wanted to build, yet God calls him a 'man after His own heart.' Maybe it's a matter of sinning while you claim to know God. David knew God, as did Moses and the Israelites; whereas Paul, when he was killing Christians, didn't know Christ. Even though his sin was very bad, God didn't punish him by not using him.

I have gotten quite a bit of literature from several different mission boards who are asking for nurses, and I will eventually write to them, but in my discouragement, I feel like I already know what their answer will be. Also, I'm beginning to see that I am not really ready to go anywhere.

To my knowledge, I don't know if I have ever won a soul to Christ, and I'm sure that would really impress a mission board! Also, I have no real Bible School training. Maybe I should just go home and get into the Discipleship Evangelism Program, and start to Bible school part time on my days off. Maybe I'm trying to run before I crawl.

Elisabeth Elliott gave another good message this morning, and I will get her tapes. I bought another copy of "Shadow Of The Almighty", and

23

asked her to sign it for me, which she did. Sure wish I could just sit and talk to her. Maybe I will write to her.

Skipped the meetings this afternoon and drove out to Three Hills Cemetery. Saw Mother Cunningham's grave, Mr. Maxwell's, and quite a few others that were familiar, though they didn't know me when we were here. Prairie has a whole big section there.

I also went to see the new hospital, as the one that Kathy, my daughter, was born in is closed and for sale. I asked about Mrs. Congo, and was told she had died a few months ago, and the home for missionary's kids, is no more. I wonder what became of their little girl with the cerebral palsy, Carol Congo.

I'm fifty-four years old, and I have never before heard a robin sing. Tonight, one was giving a beautiful God praising concert from the top of the book room building, just as God had intended him to do. How wonderful that all of creation is obedient to their Creator - and man alone is a rebel.

I saw Paul Maxwell, and gave him the 'greetings' from the Palmers. I also found out that Mr. Murray, and his daughter Rhoda, are in Japan for a year, teaching music.

How paradoxical, that here at this conference they're pleading for people to GO, and how many here are saying 'not me, Lord', and I want to go, but may never be sent. His ways are perfect, and who can know His mind?

April 19, 1985

This gem is one of Mr. Maxwell's – "And regarding clothes – some people are like birds of paradise – their feathers are worth more than their carcasses."

And, at last, the 'tea party' verse he used to say all the time.

> I had a tea party,
> This afternoon at three.
> T'was very small, three friends in all
> Just I, Myself, and Me.

It was raining when I went out this morning, and a cold wind was blowing. The rain gradually turned to snow, and on went my duffle coat and boots. I had a very nice visit with one of the graduates over a couple cups of coffee this afternoon, which was very pleasant.

Elisabeth Elliott was so good again this evening. She told about her husband Jim's death at the hands of the Auca Indians. How it was seemingly senseless, yet planned by a sovereign God. When she had learned enough of their language, she asked the young girl in the picture, taken by the men just before their deaths, about what had happened that day. The girl replied, "I told the men of the tribe, 'yes, the white men are cannibals' – so they were speared to death." When she was then asked why she had said that, she shrugged her shoulders, and said, "No reason."

But Jim Elliott has reached more for Christ in his death, than he ever could have in his life – thanks in part to his wife Elisabeth and her writing about his story.

How strange and wondrous are Your ways – past finding out, Oh, God
"He is no fool who gives what he cannot keep, to gain that which he cannot lose."

Jim Elliott

April 21, 1985   Graduation Day at Prairie

It's been so very nice to meet Susan and her friend Peggy here. Susan went out of her way to befriend me, and it's felt good to be included, and to have someone you know in the graduating class. I even went to a Three Hills home for a graduation party this afternoon.

This morning I got all ready to go to the dining room for breakfast, and couldn't get the car out of its parking spot. It was frozen in place. The front door of my motel room was also frozen shut. I finally got the car out of the parking place, backed out a way, and then got stuck in the wet snow, which had a thick layer of ice under it. There I was. I couldn't go forward or backward. A very nice man came along and rocked the car out of the spot, and I pulled up into the parking space again, and went back inside. I really didn't know what to do. It was snowing and blowing – a real blizzard! It can change in five minutes here, and it did.

It began to warm up and thaw, so about 11:30am, I tried again – and got stuck again! I don't have the right kind of tires, I was told. A woman and two girls came out, instructed me, and rocked the car out again, and I finally got going. Once I was on the highway, it was no problem. When I came back, I parked in a dry area. I was thinking of leaving after the graduation today, but decided not to. I think Susan and Peggy will go with me to Calgary tomorrow.

Last night, after Elisabeth Elliott's message, I stopped to have her sign a book she had written, and I mentioned that the last time I was here, was also the last time she was here, and that for me, it had come around full circle. Her questions to me were like arrows right to my heart. She asked if I had been a student. I said, "No, a student wife." She asked if my husband was with me. I said, "No." And the look on her face told me the rest. I came back to my room and cried, thanking God that at least HE had forgiven me! It just seems to get worse and worse. It's really discouraging to know your sin has been forgiven, but never forgotten. Is this the way it should be? I thought the sinning brother who repented was to be restored to fellowship.

I talked to the Misses Ruth and Kathleen Dearing last night. (They were music teachers at Prairie) I asked about the Congo's and they told me that the Mrs. Congo who died, was Herb Congo's mother, and that he and his wife were living in another town. Also, that their little girl, Carol, had died. They had been missionaries in Africa, and when Carol was born, and later presented with the symptoms of cerebral palsy, they were forced to leave because the natives expected them to kill her, as they would have done if the child had been theirs. That was why they had come back to Three Hills, built a huge house for missionary's children, close to Prairie's Grade School where they could go to school, and looked after about ten children of all ages. I also asked about Phyllis Wipfli, who used to baby sit for me, and she and her family also live in another town. The house she lived in, where I used to take Kathy, my two year old daughter, while I went to class, has been torn down, and is the parking lot on the corner now. Nothing stays the same, does it?

April 22, 1985

It's a beautiful day today, bright sunshine and blue sky. Had a nice drive to Calgary with Susan and Peggy, and now we're staying at a nice motel called "Ports O' Call Inn" Susan has asked me to stay another day, but I feel I must go on home. There has been somewhat of a problem between Peggy and Susan, and I have been a part of it, though not willingly or knowingly, so it seems better that I go, and relieve some of the tension. They are both very young Christians, only saved about a year and a half.

Peggy is a new diabetic at fifty-three and Susan is thirty years old. They have known each other since Susan was a baby. Peggy came to see Susan graduate, and was expecting most of Susan's time, and then I, not knowing any of this, showed up, and Susan and I just seemed to be very comfortable together, and enjoyed each other's company, while Peggy felt left out and resentful. I saw what was happening, and mentioned it to Susan. I am sorry to be the cause of anyone feeling hurt, and I pray the Lord will heal her hurt and teach her to love. How much we all need to learn to love as Jesus does.

Peggy told me today, rather proudly, that she speaks in tongues, and when I got back to my room, I began reading where I had left off, and this is what I read; "Though I speak with the tongues of men and of angels, and have not love, it profits me nothing."

Susan told me tonight that I had been like a breath of fresh air to her, for which I am thankful to the Lord. She has helped so much to soften the blows I've been getting, and it was nice to have someone to talk to about it. The Lord does know our needs, and never fails to provide for us.

May 5, 1985

I can't believe it's been two weeks since I left Prairie. Yes, I was very glad and thankful to the Lord for giving me someone to talk to there, as it was a great help to me. From what Susan said about Peggy's reaction to my being there, it's really a good thing I left when I did, and didn't stay. I have to confess that one reason I didn't want to stay, was that I was afraid Susan would ask me to pray with her, and I'm not sure I could have done that. It's so difficult for me to share my conversations with the Lord with anyone.

It's a real joy to know that someone is praying for you. I've just had the feeling that it's only me and the Lord, and no one else really cared – and you know – that's OK too. I think I need to learn to need other people. Maybe that's why I'm not needed.

Maybe I'm also afraid of failing, and not living up to what they expect of me, or what I may think they expect. So, I simply avoid any involvement just in case. Oh, the heart is deceitful and desperately wicked – who can know it?

I wanted to write down all the reasons that I am aware of, why God sent me to Prairie this spring:

1. To be an unknowing catalyst in the lives of Peggy and Susan.
2. To show me more clearly that I am far from being ready for any ministry at this time.
3. To meet Erik Bjorn, and have a part in equipping him with tapes from Grace that he has asked for.

Speaking of tapes, Marge, the number one volunteer in the 'tape shack' has quit her job, and I would love to do it. My only drawback is, I would have to miss some services from time to time when there aren't enough volunteers. Surely the Lord can provide a few people out of seven thousand people every Sunday morning! Oh, ye of little faith!

OK, I'll do it, and trust Him for the workers. And if I must sacrifice my joy in the blessing of every Sunday morning, so others might have the tapes to listen to – yes! *I'll do it gladly, Lord because I love You, my Savior, and I will do it as unto Thee!* It seems the Lord is asking me to give up what I treasure the most in my life – my Sundays at Grace, to serve Him in love, on Sundays at Grace!

Again, the paradox, but He knows, and how often what He really wants from us is, not to take away what we enjoy, but to test our willingness to loose our hold on it, if He asks it of us. How often, if we are willing to let go, He will take our empty hands and fill them to overflowing with something more wonderful than what we have let go of. *Praise the Lord, I will obey!*

May 11, 1985

Another wonderful Sunday. Much media around since the trial of Grace Church; accused of causing a young man's suicide after he had been counseled by elders here, has ended in favor of the church. They were calling it 'clergy malpractice,' but it has been dismissed on the grounds of separation of church and state.

I have been taking care of Jason in the NICU, (Newborn Intensive Care Unit) who is now 6 months old, and has never been out of this hospital. He is still on a ventilator at night, so there must be someone in the room with him all night. He is alone in the room, and no one wants to be stuck there with him in the dark all night, but I think it's great! After I get him to sleep, I pull the bedside table into the bathroom, turn on that light, open the door which screens him from the light, and I can listen to my tapes, very quietly, all night. I listen, and do counted cross stitch – and get paid for it! Only the Lord can give you a job like that! I have been so blessed listening to John's exposition of the Scripture.

In Lamentations 3:32 & 33, the Lord is speaking of His discipline in our lives, "Although God gives him grief, yet He will show compassion too, according to the greatness of His loving kindness, for He does not enjoy afflicting men, and causing sorrow." LB

It has been said that the greatest anger of God is when, He is so angry with our sin, He has abandoned us to it. If we are incurable and unteachable, we will be the objects of God's anger, when we are given up to our sin.

May 21, 1985

My Kathy is here, and it's so nice to see her again. She is a beautiful young woman, but I am so afraid for her soul. She is one to whom much light has been given, and yet no evidence of change in her life. She has been a real joy to have here. I look at her, and then at that adorable baby in the picture in the den, and it's hard to believe they are the same person. Hard to remember when she was so small. She's even getting some grey hairs! If only she would work as hard on the inner man as she does on the outer man.

I just found something I wrote when I was at Prairie. It is a note I made when a missionary from Brazil spoke.

He was telling about Brazil nuts, and he said that they grow twenty nuts together in one large round shell. It falls from the tree, but does not open. Only one of the seeds, or nuts inside, will become another Brazil nut tree; the other nineteen will provide nourishment for the one. The hard outer shell finally rots, and then roots can be put down into the earth, but until that time, the nineteen must give up being a tree, and become the sustenance for the one. The one will become a very visible tree, but the other nineteen will remain invisible, and die. Yet without them, there would be no tree. What a lesson for me!

How hard to be willing to be the invisible nourishment, that another might become the beautiful tree. It really seems as though that might be God's will for me – invisible nourishment, that another might become the visible tree. If so, praise God, I know He will enable me to do it for His glory.

As I sat down to read the other day, I asked the Lord for a word to me. I opened my Bible, and began to read Psalm 61. Verse 6 reads, "You will give me added years of life, as rich and full as those of many generations all packed into one." LB

Oh, what a wave of sudden insight went over me, and I asked, "Oh, Lord, is that for me?" I hope he was saying that the years left to me will be double in richness and fullness in service for Him, making up for some of the wasted years – as many generations packed into one. It really blessed my heart, and I rejoiced to hear my Lord speak just to me, when I needed some encouragement.

May 27, 1985   Memorial Day

My mom, and my daughter Kathy went to Tonopah for the weekend, but I had to work Saturday night. It was my fourth twelve hour shift in a row, and I was tired. I prayed, believing it to be God's will, that He would give me strength to make it to church on Sunday morning. I hate to work on Saturday night, as it makes Sunday so difficult.

But, again, I asked for God to use me, and I want to be poured out for Him; and then when He does, I find myself either collapsing, or complaining. How weak I am!

"Oh, Savior, how tired you must have been in your humanity, and yet how willing you were to pour out your life in love for us."

At work, I was able to have a time to talk to Rex, a young Japanese respiratory therapist, who has found the Lord, while his whole family remains Buddhist, and are persecuting him for his stand. I try to encourage him to remain faithful, and to pray for his family. I also had an opportunity to talk to Julie. She says she is a Christian, but she is unmarried, and pregnant for the second time. I spoke to her several months ago about living for the Lord, but then her boy friend came back, and now she is pregnant again. I felt very bad about it, and thought of how we must break the heart of our loving Lord when we live only for ourselves as we do. I certainly can't point a finger at anyone, but if it grieves me, how much more must it grieve Him?

Sunday morning after work, I was amazed, I really felt good! Why are we amazed when we receive what we have asked for? Such unbelievable unbelief! It was Marge's last day, and she gave me her key to the Tape Shack. She has done a wonderful job, but has become unhappy and resentful, and has felt unappreciated! It's sad when we feel we must be appreciated for what we do for Christ.

I am so grateful to the Lord for giving me this marvelous opportunity for a ministry at Grace. I keep thinking about what John said about who the Lord looks for when he needs someone for a job. It's the busy people, not those sitting and waiting. I want to be busy for Him!

I went home, took a three hour nap, and went back for the evening service, where Chris Mueller had a good message on the sovereignty of God.

Today (Monday) I am alone, and it's been a good day. I've listened to several tapes, and on one of them, John read a poem from his grandfather's Bible, written by Martha Snell Nicholson. It fit so well, I wrote it down in my Bible. It sort of parallels my life.

"When I stand at the Judgment seat of Christ,
And He shows me His plan for me;
The plan of my life as it might have been, and
I see how I blocked Him here, and checked Him there,
And would not yield my will;
Will there be grief in my Savior's eyes,
Grief, though He loves me still?
You see, He would have me rich, and I stand there poor,
Stripped of all but His grace,
While memory runs, like a haunted thing,
Down a path that I can't retrace.
My desolate heart will surely break,
With tears I cannot shed,
I will cover my face with my empty hands,
I will bow my uncrowned head.
Oh, Lord of the years that are left to me,
I give them to Thine hand;
Take me, break me, mold me
To the pattern Thou hast planned.

Martha Snell Nicholson

Being broken hurts, but that hurt is joyous compared to the pain of having to cover my face with my empty hands in His presence! Can it be that He will still use me? How can He be so patient and merciful? I deserve nothing but death, and He has given me life! *"Oh, Savior, teach me to follow hard after Thee!"*

I have gone to the Master's College, and asked for a catalog. I hope it will come soon. I'm still thinking and praying about Bible School. The Master's College would be nice as it's so close to home, yet I think of Prairie and how nice it would be to have a whole year of just studying God's Word in a cozy little room – marvelous!

And then I think, no mission board will take me – yet, our God is able! I can't give up. He must have some place for me. Perhaps, after the breaking and molding, then, He will show me His plan; when I am ready, and not before. *"Help me, Lord, to not run before You, there are so many pit-falls! Help me to stay behind You, my Shepherd, so I can follow where You are leading."*

I know that real happiness lies only in obedience. I want to make my list here of those who were refused the desire of their hearts because of their sin.

1. Moses – not allowed to enter into the Promised Land.
2. A whole generation of Israelites because they complained, and refused to obey.
3. David – not allowed to build the Temple.
4. Esau – not allowed to have his birthright back – though he repented with tears.
5. The runner in the race- not allowed to run but, set aside, out of the way of the other runners.

How can I be so bold as to think I might escape the consequences of sin, and be allowed to do what I want so much to do? Is this the final answer, or am I only looking at one side of a question?

August 14, 1985

There is so much to write, I don't know where to begin. It seems in God's timing the waiting may be over. I must back up to the day at Family Camp when I talked with Monnie Brewer. I explained my experience with Wycliffe, and he gave me some addresses to write to; Intercristo, Medical Ambassadors, and one other, similar to Intercristo.

I wrote to them all, and soon received answers from them all. Intercristo's response was a long list of organizations looking for Christian nurses, but there was nothing there for me. Medical Ambassadors had been one of the speakers at one of the mission's meetings at Prairie, but I had left early, as it just didn't seem to be anything for me, but their response to my letter of inquiry was very nice, and at the bottom of it, before he signed his name, Dr. Benson said, "Let me encourage you with this significant statement: 'God will not put a desire in your heart, unless He intends to fulfill it.'" The very words that both Susan first, and then John had said to me. Here they were again – same words – for the third time! John has always said that when God repeats something, He's very serious about it, and we'd better listen real close! So – I read all the literature they sent to me, and in it was a note about a Pediatric clinic, and nutrition center in Cap-Haitien, Haiti. It is run by two American nurses, and they were praying for a third nurse to help them. He felt that my qualifications were just what they needed. Then He asked, "Would you be interested?"

Would I be interested?!!

Praise the Lord! I really liked the definition, the objectives, the methodology, and the goals of the organization, so, I thought – after prayer – why not? I sent for an application and statement of faith. When they came, I filled them out, being very thankful that it didn't require my writing down all of my past. It simply asked, married, single, or divorced? I checked divorced, and that was all.

I also said, that, yes, I would be interested in Haiti. Then I signed the statement of faith, and sent it all back They had told me it would be two to three weeks before I would hear from them, so I settled down to wait. About a week later, I received a letter from Dr. Benson, stating he had received my application, and that I certainly was eligible, and yes, they definitely had a place for me in Haiti!

The door, so long being knocked upon, was actually beginning to open! Dr. Benson asked that I make plans to come to Modesto, where they were located, for an interview.

Now, to show again how our God is indeed Sovereign God, little things had happened. My schedule at work had been changed, much to my upset, and now I have to work Monday, Tuesday, and Wednesday one week, and Thursday, Friday, and Saturday, the next week. This gives me three days off one week, and five the next. After I had received this last letter, I looked to see when I had the next five days off, so I could drive to Modesto. It fell on the tenth through the fourteenth, so, I phoned Dr. Benson, and told him I would come on the twelfth and thirteenth, and he said that was fine. (I had signed up for Discipleship Evangelism at Grace, and it begins next Monday, for a sixteen week commitment, so this was the only time I could have gone.)

Then, I phoned Monnie Brewer to tell him what was happening, and that I really wanted to have Grace Church behind me, not financially, necessarily, but to know that the elders would pray for me, know I was out there, and remember me before the Lord. This, I now found presented a problem.

Grace Church has a very good program designed to equip those going to the mission field, and I didn't know much about it. I had been to the missions meetings, but never really knew what they were talking about, when they talked about Stage 1, Stage 2, etc. Monnie told me, that to be supported by Grace Church, I needed to get into this program so that the elders could get to know me, in order to feel responsible for me, and that this takes time. Up to five years!

Then, he also said that it could be much shorter if God should lay me on the hearts of the elders that they could feel I should go sooner.

I was very confused and upset. I felt that I had done what Monnie had told me to do, and now it seems, it was maybe the wrong thing. I agreed that he was right, and reasonable, but, now, I don't know what to do. I decided to call Dr. Benson, and tell him, and see if he still wanted me to come to Modesto. I tried four times. Three times, no one answered, and the fourth time, I just didn't feel I could do it, and put the phone down. I didn't try again, but I felt that I should go, that this was God's directive. I felt very much at peace when I drove up on Monday morning. I even wore a dress. How good the Lord is! He has led me every step of the way – even to the smallest detail. He doesn't forget anything.

August 19, 1985

It was an exciting and blessed time. I talked to Dr. Benson and his wife, Lou while they finished their lunch. Then Dick Hillis came and spoke to me. I was taken to the Medical Ambassador's office, where I met Nancy. From there we went to the home of Joyce and Jason Johnson, where I was left. Jason drove me back, later, to the Benson's where dinner was waiting.

Then, the Fulfer's came over. He is an attorney and a board member. Such delightful, and wonderful Christian people, and the really marvelous thing is they all – independently - said, the past is past, and it's where you are now, that's important! Even Dick Hillis said that, much to Dr. Benson's surprise.

Praise the Lord! He is an overcoming God! Perhaps He will send me out . They were even glad that I wanted Grace Church behind me, and glad that I was going into the 16 weeks of Discipleship Evangelism there.

All of this happened on Monday. On Tuesday morning, I talked some more with Dr. Benson, and then I left to drive home about 1:30 – feeling absolutely overjoyed – and wiped out!

Now, it will be grand to see how the Lord will work it all out. He is able – if I am to go to Haiti – to tell the elders that I am ready, and that it is the Lord's will for me to go as a part of, and sent from, Grace Church. I really believe that even as He has over ruled my past, He is able to work in the hearts of the elders of Grace. Amen!

Tonight I worked with a Philippino girl by the unbelievable name of Primrose. She heard someone asking me questions about my trip to Modesto, so when we were alone, she began asking me questions. I was able to talk to her about the Lord, the plan of salvation, marriage, divorce, Heaven, and more that I can't remember. It lasted for nearly the whole twelve hours. It was wonderful! Just the two of us in the Preemie Room, with only four babies to care for. She says she is a born again Christian, and was so receptive to Scripture.

I praise the Lord for such a great opportunity to be a witness for Him. It's such a joy to be able to spend so much time talking about the things of the Lord. I know that is not what the hospital pays me to do, but, all of that got done as well.

It's amazing to me to see how the Lord has narrowed my scope, and at the same time, enlarged my heart and my vision. I feel like I have heavenly blinders on, and can no longer see what goes on around me. Nothing in the news, TV, magazines, books or pastimes seems to be important anymore. All I am interested in is to read, see, or talk about the things of the Lord. At the same time my heart aches more and more, for those around me, for whom all of these other things are so important. Even my bookshelf tells the story.

When I first came to my mom's two years ago, the bookshelf was filled with gothic romances, and trashy novels. They have gradually been replaced with tapes, and with books on missions and missionaries, Bible study guides, and commentaries. The novels are gone! Also, when I came, my prime interest was doll making. They, too, have been replaced with the time taken up with the things of the Lord. He is SO good!

I thought it would be painful to let go of the things I really enjoyed, but they seem to have just fallen away without any effort on my part at all. He has done it with His infinite tenderness and love. I have only ONE love now. He alone is the joy of my heart, nothing else can compare. This world has nothing to offer me that could begin to compare with my wonderful Savior. And yet, I know that I have not 'arrived'. He has a lot more work to do on me. I long to be so yielded to Him, and to be used that He might be glorified.

Here is another of God's providential happenings, a television program on Haiti. I'm falling in love with the people of Haiti after seeing that program. It's a feeling that only God could give. I had no deep longing in my heart for Haiti. I really didn't even know where Haiti was! The more I hear and see, the more I'm hoping that God will send me there. These may be what one of the elders, calls 'sealing circumstances' in knowing God's will. These things happening in the hearts of those concerned and involved with my quest, are things that must be given by God, as they are impossible to work up on your own.

August 27, 1985

The hospital called me today and asked if I could work days today. I couldn't really think of any reason why I couldn't, so today found me again in the NICU. It's always so good to know that my gracious Shepherd always goes before this poor sheep, and I'm always so eager to see what He will do, especially in different circumstances, and with different people. I will be working with the day people instead of my usual night folks.

I was assigned two sweet uncomplicated babies, one of which was to go back to Santa Barbara today, back to the hospital he was transported from. I really didn't want to take a four and a half hour ambulance ride in this heat, but I said I would go. I thought that the Respiratory Therapist that would go with us would be a young Philippino, who is new on the unit. Then to my surprise and delight, I found it would be a wonderful, mature Christian young man that I admire. His work for the Lord is very unusual, and he really loves the Lord. So – for three and a half hours we talked in the back of the ambulance, while our patient slept peacefully.

I told him about Haiti, and was glad to hear him reinforce the fact that we don't want to run ahead of the Lord, but need to wait for Him to bring His plan to it's fulfillment. He said that it was very important for me to have the elders of Grace behind me, praying for me, and holding me up before the Lord. I was glad to hear him say that.

When I got home, my mom told me that I'd had a phone call from a nurse in Haiti! It was Diana, from the Medical Ambassador's clinic. I also had a letter from Dr. Benson. He said that he'd gotten back from Haiti, and that Diana was going to write a letter to me – and here she was, calling me! She called again about 8:30pm, and it was good to talk to her, but I was glad that the Lord had impressed on me again today, that it must be in His way, and in His time. If that hadn't happened, after listening to her plea for me to come soon, I probably would have gone tomorrow! How exciting to see our living God, stooping down to us from Heaven to direct even the smallest detail of our lives when they are given over to Him. Praise the Lord!

September 9, 1985

Praises to our Savior King! Today was such a special Sunday. John's morning message was so good, and then – so special – the inauguration of John as President of The Master's College. Wonderful music, lots of impressive college gowns, robes, and great speakers. Dr. Sweeting, the President of Moody Bible Institute, and the former President of the Master's College. He was wonderful – must have been in his eighties or nineties – had to be helped up to the podium by the Associated Student body President.

John spoke only a bit, but it's so marvelous to hear him say, how often he looks around and doesn't know why God is doing what He is doing, or why God is using him. He says he's amazed, and feels like he is looking on as a spectator – not really knowing what's happening. I just pray that God will always keep him as humble and true to the calling God has given him.

Every time I re-read this, I marvel anew at the way God works in our lives. I was reading through Jeremiah, and the analogy of the potter and the clay was so good! Then, the next issue of a small Christian magazine had an article on these very verses, and brought out some wonderful new thoughts.

God, of course, is the Potter, and we are the clay. The beauty of His vessels comes from His heart and His hands, not from some privileged environment. Left to itself, the clay would forever remain formless, and useless. It can not know the Potter's mind, or direct the Potter's hands.

The potter's wheel is our round of everyday life. The clay must remain one with the turning disc, for as long as the work needs to continue. Only the finished product would be separated from the Potter's wheel, now ready to be used.

At times, the pressure of His fingers against the clay seems hard enough to crush the forming vessel, yet that will never happen. At other times, the pressure seems too slight to accomplish anything – yet it is always enough to accomplish exactly the design He has for that vessel. The Potter's power over the clay, is God's right to deal with His universe as He wills. He does not deal capriciously with the clay at His disposal, but forms it according to His wise and eternal purpose.

The Divine Potter can not mold the human clay apart from the wheel of circumstance which He has ordained. It is a gradual process, and there are no shortcuts in His bringing us to completion. When the vessel is marred, or spoiled, or broken, it is not BY the Potter's hand, but IN His hand. The vessel may have broken, but it was still in the Potter's hand. As He applied the necessary pressure to mold the vessel, He knew that it must conform to His design, or crumble.

Though we may fall apart from the pressure in our lives, we are still in the Potter's hands, and He intends to do a reconstruction job – not a mending – but a whole new vessel, beginning with a second kneading of the lump. We may be broken, but we are never lost to Him! God still has His plan, regardless of what has happened along the way. It is amazing what God can do with broken vessels – providing He is given all the pieces. God never loses His purpose for us, nor His ability to accomplish His purpose.

Just as it takes a miracle of Divine grace to redeem the lost, so it takes a miracle of Divine grace to make anew the redeemed life that has fallen in carnal disobedience.

God loves to do both miracles! The important thing is not what we have been, or what we are now, but what we are becoming in His hands. He will do this for us, not that we might enjoy being a beautiful or useful vessel, but rather because, in so re-making a spoiled vessel – He receives what is due Him – glory! And that is as it should be!

What a wonderful, encouraging analogy for those of us who once were spoiled or marred vessels. I believe that God is in the process of re-making me. It is a gradual process, requiring me to learn patience, but the Potter is the Master Craftsman, who never makes a mistake!

"But we have this treasure in earthen vessels, that the Excellency of the Power may be of God, and not of us."
II Corinthians 4:7 KJV

December 10, 1985

Even though I wish I could leave for Haiti tomorrow, I know that this is not His plan for me now. I have been reading about J.O. Fraser of Lisu Land, and he said something that put into words how I feel about going anywhere, only, with the consent and blessing of the elders at Grace. Fraser said that he was, " . . . the hand stretching, and reaching out to the Lisu people, but a hand can not be cut off from the body, or it will die. This is how I feel about Grace Church, they must be the body, giving life and support to me, the hand. I can't cut myself off, and go on my own strength. I would not be able to function at all, but would be a dead hand, and useless.

I pray that Diana and Flo in Haiti, and Dr. Benson in Modesto, will be able to see this as I do, and be willing to patiently wait, and hope. God is never in a hurry, and His plan is best, the only plan that will work, and bring Him glory. And that's the real purpose of our lives anyway, isn't it? Not that I go to Haiti, not that Haitian babies get fed and cared for, not even that those same Haitians hear the Good News, but that God will be glorified in it all – from the remaking of the marred vessel, to the daily use of it. Amen!

I forgot to mention something else to praise and thank the Lord for in everything. My car was broken into Friday night in the parking structure of the hospital. My radio and speakers were stolen. One of John's tapes was in the tape deck, and I pray that whoever took my radio will listen to the tape, be convicted of their sin, and come to the Lord.

December 17, 1985

Three months have gone by since I last wrote in this, partly due to some discouragement on my part, plus, nothing of any great moment has happened. I have finished my 16 weeks of Discipleship Evangelism, and it was worth all of the effort to finish it. I have never felt such negative opposition to anything before. Satan really didn't want me to finish this, knowing that when I did, I would have another tool to use in winning souls to the Lord, and away from the evil one.

I had the opportunity to use this tool with a young woman, here in the hospital, who was anorexic, and also bi-polar. I knew I shouldn't be taking the time when I was at work to talk to her, so I went to see her on two different Sundays, and spent about an hour and a half each time with her. Then I found out it was against hospital policy for me to even befriend her.

I was sent to the Nursing Director of the hospital, where I was told I could be terminated if I persisted. The girl is so controlled by her sickness that she fears everything. She told me she is afraid to become a Christian because she is afraid of what satan will do to her. I have told her that without Christ, she has no defense, but all she does is cry and say, "I'm so afraid." Poor, poor child, she was soon sent to another facility when her insurance wouldn't pay anymore.

Tomorrow I will go and talk to Anthony Shepherd, an elder at Grace Church. Al Mount, another elder in the Outreach Department asked me to talk to him about my divorces, so the elders would not be surprised by them, if I ever came up before them. I don't really want to talk about it – I wish I could just bury it all in the depths of the sea, never to be brought up again! But, God knows the way I take – the beginning and the end – and all of it is in His hands.

The Potter can still make a vessel of beauty and usefulness of my life, not because of anything I am – I am only the clay, but because it will be to His glory to do it. What a miracle, for Him to take a ruined vessel, and not mend it, but remake it!

I have begun to wonder if the Lord might keep me here. I can see my mother going down hill, physically. Sunday, she began complaining that something had happened to her eyes, but the eye doctor said nothing was wrong with them, that it might have been a transient ischemic attack (TIA) though her blood pressure was not too high today, it might have been on that day. Sometimes I feel that I am also becoming a hindrance to her independence, because when I am here, she is inclined to look to me for things that she is quite capable of doing for herself, but my first obligation is to look after her. The Lord knows this, too, and it is in His tender hands. I am willing to go, or to stay, as He wills, and He is leading the way, praise His wonderful Name!

December 18, 1985

At last, I have met and talked with Anthony Shepherd. What a kind and sensitive man he is. I was really a little afraid at first, but he was very easy to talk to, though I think I listened more than I talked.

In essence, what he told me was, it was very important where I was now, not so much of where I had been in my past. Obedience to the leading of the Lord was what was essential now. I enjoyed him very much, and was in his office for two hours. I felt that he was satisfied with where I am, and he encouraged me by asking me to stop and see him again, or writing to tell him how the Lord was leading in my life. He said he was excited, and was eager to hear about it.

Everything that he suggested I do, I have been doing. The heart is so deceitful, and I must ask the Lord to show me if I am deceiving myself about my desire for service, and check my motives. He was ready to end our conversation after I told him about my first two husbands, and I sat there thinking – should I leave him thinking there were only two, or should I tell him about the others as well? I wanted to be open and honest, and put it all out there, so I said, " I haven't finished yet," and went on. I feel better about it now, and I hope he knows how much I sorrow over the sins of the past. I know the blood of Christ covers even that, and gives to me a cleanness possible only in Him. I have exchanged my ugly life for His righteous and beautiful life, and thank God, that is how He sees me now, perfect in Him!

I've been feeling lately as though I am bogging down, and not really growing with the joy and enthusiasm I had. I guess this is common, but I don't like it. I pray that God will build a great fire under me, and get me moving upward again. George Whitfield said, "Lord, when you see me nestling down, put a thorn in my nest!" Maybe that's what I need, a thorn in my nest.

I've been thinking of starting a Bible study here in Friendly Valley for some of the ladies, but I don't have any idea how to go about it, or where to start. One thing I remember being said today; was that ignorance is no excuse for sin. It was for sins done in ignorance that atonement was made by the Levitical priests. I hadn't realized this, but, of course, willful sin was atoned for by punishment in that time. How blessed are we in this age of grace – I would be dead otherwise!

"Thank You, Gracious Father, for Your warm loving encouragement today."

December 29, 1985

Christmas and a New Year – one is past, and the other nearly here. How fast this year has flown! It's been a great year of growing in the Lord – ever striving, never arriving!

Yesterday, I received a phone call from Flo Hachmier, one of the nurses in Haiti, who is there under Medical Ambassadors. She is in her seventies and said the Lord didn't call her until she was 60. She told me a lot about Haiti, and now I am even more eager to go and work there. She said she rents a three bedroom, two bath house, with one of the few bath tubs in Haiti, and she said I could have one of the bedrooms. It sounds so wonderful! (I was expecting a tiny shack, which would have been OK.) She also told me about the trips they take into the mountains for clinics, so I guess I had better get out and start walking to get into shape so I can keep up!

I really need more discipline in my life. Right now, I'd be a pretty sorry soldier or athlete – too much chocolate and too little exercise. Flo also told me she will be starting language study in March. It will be a six week, one on one course, and they were hoping I could be there in time to do it with her. I am so excited! I just pray that the Lord will send me!

Flo also told me that there have been some riots, and unrest in several of the cities there, but that doesn't frighten me. I'd rather be in the middle of a revolution – in His will – than be secure in my own bed at home – out of His will! I long to give my life in His service, and I have given some thought about prisons, firing squads, torture, and terrible things like this, and I have wondered if I could stand firm in Christ, and not deny my Lord. I think most Christians wonder about this at some time in their life. There is such unrest in the world today, and in this blessed country, we live in such isolated comfort with our fat stomachs and flabby muscles. We can not imagine what it is like to be really hungry, or cold, or sick, or hurting, and have no where to go for help of any kind. We simply have no idea what millions of people are suffering today, and how they are in desperate need of someone to care for them and their needs.

I am afraid for America. God has said, "To whom much is given, much shall be required." We will answer for our sins of selfishness as individuals, and as a nation. God will require a just judgment on our stewardship of the resources He has so bountifully given us. I wonder how it will be when the Lord will call me home. I just thank Him that He has promised that I will share His home for eternity, so it doesn't matter how, or when, He may call me. Amen!

January 1, 1986

"You have done so much for me, Oh, Lord. No wonder I am glad! I sing for joy!"

Psalm 92:4 LB

My heart is one with David tonight as I think back over the past year, and see how the Lord has worked in my life. I am closer to what I should be, but I am still far from what He would have me be – more like the Savior. He is not finished with me yet, and I am looking forward to this year, and wonder what my life will be.

We had our watch night service at Grace Church tonight, and as always, it was such a blessing! It is beyond everyone's wildest dreams the way God is moving there, and to have even a small (very small) part of what is happening is very exciting. Exciting to see God at work, in His sovereignty, bringing everything together for His glory!

When I got home, it was 1:15am. I just wanted to thank Him, and get into my bed. I decided to read a small portion, and when I opened my Bible, it opened to Psalm 92. I began to read and pray, and then I realized that it was my favorite Psalm, the one that says in verses 12- 15, "But the godly shall flourish like palm trees, and grow tall like the cedars of Lebanon, for they are transplanted into the Lord's own garden, and are under His personal care. Even in old age they will still produce fruit and be vital and green. This honors the Lord, and exhibits His faithful care. He is my shelter. There is nothing but goodness in Him!" LB

Again, I am claiming these verses as God's promises to me. That, as I possess the righteousness of Christ, I shall flourish and grow tall in Him. He has transplanted me from the world's garden into His own garden, where He is the gardener, and will care for me personally – feeding and pruning as necessary, so that I will produce fruit, even in old age, and still be vital and green. And why? Not that I might be a thing of beauty, or that the fruit I produce will make me more valuable, but because it will honor and glorify Him – the husbandman, the gardener. The plant with its' green leaves and fruit is a reflection of the gardener's tender loving care, without which it would die.

I long with all my being, to be a fruitful plant that will bring honor to the Lord. I pray that this year will be one of His feeding, and my growing; His pruning, and my bearing more fruit to His glory. Maybe in Haiti, maybe not, but wherever, may He be glorified, and may I be all that He has created me to be for Him!

January 2, 1986

Today is Tina's birthday – she's all of four years old, and such a darling little thing, who goes around singing in a tiny little voice all the time. May our blessed Lord be the joy of her life!

I feel like a total failure today. I got up at 4:30am, and went to Grace Church, where everyone was waiting to go to the conference on Missionary Preparation, at UCLA. We drove down, and began registering people. I was helping with the meal ticket envelopes. As it began to get on toward time for the first session, we were told we'd better hurry. No one had told us it was a 15 minute hike down hill, and then up hill to the auditorium. It was easy going down hill. We got there late, it was very warm in the room, and my throat was beginning to feel swollen and scratchy. We sat toward the back, and as the first speaker began to speak, – I started to fade. I more or less slept through the first speaker, and when he finished, they gave us a break. I found a coffee machine and though it tasted pretty good, it didn't do much for my fuzzy head and weak knees. I managed to stay a bit more awake through the second speaker, and then it was lunch time. We retraced our steps to the dorm, and by the time I pulled my poor body up that last step, I knew I'd never make that same trip two more times that day! Then, I thought, maybe after some food, I'd feel better. I stood for twenty minutes in line, got some food, stood in some more lines (no drinks of any kind) – very unorganized – sat down to eat, and everything was cold! The reason I feel like such a failure is, at this point, I decided to go home. It all seemed really pointless in the light of the need in Haiti, and I really didn't feel well at all, so, I went home. Three days pay lost, plus $107.00 paid out, for nothing.

All the way home I wondered if I was a quitter, and too soft for the mission field. I believe I could do it if it was for something I believed in, but for that! It just really wasn't worth it. I hope I have not been disobedient to the Lord. I say, "at any cost", but do I really mean it?

"Please teach me Lord, what it means to say, at any cost, and really mean it."

January 3, 1986

I Got up this morning feeling much better; sat and read <u>The Seduction of Christianity,</u> by Dave Hunt for a couple of hours, and then decided to take a shower and get dressed. As I was going toward the bathroom, I thought about the program at UCLA that I was supposed to be participating in, and I looked at the schedule again.

I decided to go to the workshops. I got there in time for the 'Tentmaker's' talk, which was a very good presentation of language and culture learning by a BIOLA teacher named Lingenfelter, who had been a missionary on the island of Yap. Then I went to Al Mount's talk on, "Things I Wish I'd Learned Before I Went" session. All of them were good, and the walk back and forth was invigorating. I am listening again to John's tapes on the Charismatics. They are so good, and tonight I talked to my cousin Denny, and discovered that he goes to a Pentecostal church that speaks in tongues, so I will plan to send him the album.

I'm glad I was able to go back and get in on some more of the conference. There were some very good things talked about in all three sessions, and I've got some good notes. Well, praise the Lord, He is so good. Every good gift I have , I have from His hand, and by His grace.

January 12, 1986

"Ah, Lord God! Behold Thou hast made the heaven and the earth by Thy great power and outstretched arm, and there is nothing too difficult for Thee!"

Jeremiah 32: 17 KJV

I am so excited tonight, I'm not sure I'll be able to sleep. At the missions meeting today, I went to the Outreach Office to take back a book that someone had found for me – the last one on the Stage One list! Al Mount was there, and said he'd just gotten back from a retreat for the elders, and he said that my name had come up. Then someone told me later, that some good things had been said about me there. How my heart is rejoicing tonight, and how good the Father is to His children! How thrilling it is to wait on the Lord, and watch Him do all the things that I, in my human frailty, can not do. I belong to the Sovereign God of the universe, and He is truly able to move mountains if He chooses, and to remove the obstacles in the pathway that He has chosen for His child.

How can we be anxious or fearful, when our Shepherd lovingly walks before us, leading us? I know that God is in control of my life, and He is giving me the grace to be obedient in everything. Praise His name! I even walked past the chocolate cookies I dearly love today, and didn't buy any. I wasn't sure I could really do it, but I must gain the control over my body. I am also out walking every day I'm off, and at work, I try to go up and down the stairs at least once. I'm trying to get myself in shape to hike into the mountain villages that Flo was telling me about. I wouldn't make it a mile in the shape I'm in right now.

The Lord has spoken to me twice about the chocolate. One evening service, John was mentioning those who let various things rule their lives, and I was sitting there so smugly, since none of it was hitting me. Suddenly, he let fly the arrow that zinged me! "Would you believe," he said, "that some people HAVE to have their chocolate!"

Wow! Ouch! He got me! Then in another message at the Master's College – same thing again. I have really had a battle, but I will not be brought into subjection to something like this, and in Haiti, I'll be thankful just for food – so, "Good bye chocolate!"

Why is it the dumb little things in our lives that seem to give us such big problems? The victory is ours in Christ, for the battle has already been won for us, and the enemy is under His feet. In Romans 16:20, it says that God will bruise Satan under OUR feet shortly. Praise the Lord ! What a gracious God we serve, who is willing to share His love, and His work with people like us.

January 14, 1986

How exciting to see God at work. How He stoops to move one grain of sand – me; how unworthy I am of all the wonders He has done, just to give me the joy of serving Him!

I didn't know it, but Dr. Benson told me that they had had a prayer meeting on Saturday – the day the elders were on retreat, and were discussing me, and they – Dr. Benson and group, were praying for me at the same time. Also, I had finished Stage one of the preparation program at Grace Church, and I had made an appointment with Al Mount to find out what I needed to do next, and before I even knew about the elder's retreat, Al told them – on faith, he said – without really knowing it, that I had completed Stage one. God's timing is perfect! My talk with Anthony Shepherd was also mentioned, so I presume they now know all there is to know about me, except - why I want to go to Haiti.

I am to go before the selection committee on February fifth, at 7:15am to give them my reason for wanting to go to Haiti. Praise the Lord! He is able. His hand is outstretched to me, and He is moving in my life. What a joy, what a miracle that the Creator of all, would stoop to listen to the cry of my heart, and answer me! What a great and glorious God is this God, there is none like Him!

January 29, 1986

I have been listening to a tape on Matthew 2:1, about the Magi. What an awesome thing to see how God is in control of history – it truly is His story!

How the Magi, six hundred years before Christ was born, were brought into contact with Daniel, and there came to know about the true and living God, and about the prophecies of the coming King.

Then, six hundred years later, they came seeking the Promised One, and found Him, lying in a manger. Amazing, how the first to acknowledge Him as King, were the ancient king-makers from the east, Gentiles, not even His own people. What a great truth!

I sat in on the Outreach council tonight – rather interesting. What a sweet young man Tim Brannigan is. I can see why John is discipling him. I left rather early to go home from an Outreach meeting, at 9pm. The last meeting, it was mid-night when they finished.

I talked earlier with Dr. Benson, and he told me that there is a lot of unrest in Haiti. An insurrection has caused the schools to be closed by the President, so there is no language school for the present, at least no dates for me to give to the selection committee. It's just so exciting to see God's hand in it all. I don't have a clue how He is leading at this point, but I know He is. If He can move in history as He has – can I have any doubt as to what He is able to do? None! He is still the God of all the ages, and He is still in control! And I am still led by His own omnipotent hand – how glorious and how simple; all I have to do is whatever He says to do, and follow where He leads, knowing, that as a loving father leads his little child around the dangers, and over the hard places, even so, my Heavenly Father in love, leads me.

February 11, 1986

It's been quite awhile since I've opened this, and much has happened. God is so obviously working in my life, it is beyond imagining – just as His word says – above and beyond all that we can ask or think!

On February fifth, I went before a selection committee of eight or more men, (I can't remember, I was so nervous.) I was introduced all around, and then Al asked me to give a short testimony, and tell them about the work in Haiti, which I did. They then asked me questions which I tried to answer. When they were finished with their questions, they asked me to leave, and wait for their decision.

I went out and prayed that the Holy Spirit would give them wisdom, that His perfect will for many lives might be done. I waited, for what seemed like hours, trying not to look apprehensive or worried, which I really wasn't, but it did seem like forever before they finally came out. Al asked me to come up to his office for a few minutes, and for a minute I thought the answer must be, "No", but on the way up the stairs he told me they had been favorable!

Now, the problem is - the situation in Haiti. It has worsened, and the Dictator, Papa Doc Duvalier and his fancy wife, crept out of the country under cover of darkness, and fled to France, taking all of the country's money with them. No country wants them on a permanent basis. The people of Haiti are behaving like any who have been denied even the barest essentials of life, in subjection so brutal, and they are smashing everything, and anything to do with him. He has bled the country dry, then gathered it all up, and run away with what rightly belongs to the people. You can be sure that God will judge him for his wickedness. Now, it remains to be seen what will happen there, as they try to form a new government.

How exciting to know that it is God who puts men in power, and brings them down, so I will just wait on His time. They will not let me go there as long as there are riots and unrest, so I pray that all will end soon, and a good government will take over.

The plan at this point is for me to work until April 15, and then go to Haiti for private language tutoring for six weeks, then go to Cap-Haitien, and spend two weeks in the clinic. All of this as a taste to see if I can do it, and if I will fit in. Then I would come home for two to three weeks of missionary internship at a special program at the Master's College (five minutes from home.)

I am so excited I can hardly stand it. Praise the Lord!!! It's getting closer, and is finally becoming a reality. I know that the God who has brought me this far, will not quit now, but will bring His plan to perfection, just as He has promised in His word – for His name's sake!

Al called Dr. Benson while I was in his office, and Dr. Benson was pleased, and as always, gracious and submissive in his reply to the plan laid out before him by Al. I then talked to Dr. Benson, and he said it looks like August or September before I can be there to stay. It's been a little more than a year of waiting, but I have learned so much in this year, and to God, in His economy, what is a year! He is in control! Amen!

February 26, 1986

Two weeks have passed since 'Baby Doc Duvalier' left Haiti, and there is no more news on TV about the situation in Haiti. God is the One who sets up and brings down those in power, and in the last two weeks, He has brought two men down, Duvalier in Haiti, and Marcos in the Philippines. Now it remains to be seen who He will set up in their places. It's comforting to know that none of this 'just happens', but all is a part of God's plan.

I went to the baptism service this evening, and it was inspiring, as always. Then I went to another Outreach meeting from 8:30 until 12 midnight.

As I was talking to Al Mount, he told me he had written to Dr. Benson, and that what was mentioned at the selection committee about the church not giving me any financial support was a misunderstanding, and that there will be some support for me from Grace Church. Praise the Lord! Al even said it was already in the budget. I knew that God would do for me whatever I needed, just as He has been doing all along. Money was no problem, and He has proved that! Also, two girls at work said they would like to have a part in this ministry as well. Then I got a phone call from an old neighbor that I haven't seen or heard from in quite a few years, and she wants to have a part. Amazing!!

I read an interesting letter from Dr. Al Warren, who was an elder at Grace, and is now a dentist in Haiti. He'd written to let Monnie, and the church, know that he and his family in Port-au- Prince were OK, and in no danger. He also mentioned something interesting that I hadn't thought about before. He feels that the upper class of Haiti is a forgotten people when it comes to being reached with the Gospel. Missionaries all come to reach the poor people, but seem to have forgotten about the rich folks. (I thought all the rich folk had left with Duvalier.)

Dr. Warren said that the upper class is religious, and not as involved in Voodoo, but they are just as lost with out Christ, as the poor people are. Also, they speak English, which makes the work easier. I must write to Dr. Warren soon.

I just opened my Bible to these wonderful verses in Isaiah;

"The Lord God has given me His words of wisdom so that I may know what I should say to all these weary ones. Morning by morning He wakens me and opens my understanding to His will.

Because the Lord God helps me, I will not be dismayed; therefore, I have set my face like flint to do His will, and I know that I will triumph."

Isaiah 50: 4 and 7 LB

March 26, 1986

Tonight, I am the weary one, weary in trying to understand just which direction the Lord would have me to go. Medical Ambassadors is getting impatient, and I can't blame them, looking at the situation from their point of view. Diana, who was responsible for the clinic under Medical Ambassadors, has left, and now Flo is there alone. They have been waiting for me for nine months, and I still can't give them a definite date. I had hoped it would be the end of this month, but now I'm not sure.

First, I was to go for six weeks, and then come back. Then, it was three weeks, but today, I was told three months, which would eliminate the Master's College Missionary Internment Program in May, and tonight, Monnie again said that he really wanted me to go to that. I really don't know – but I know the Lord knows!

Dr. Benson has made a reservation for me on Agape Flights for the thirtieth of April, and I am very confused. To add to all of that, I have given the hospital my resignation, and my last day there is to be the eleventh of April, plus I have bought a ticket to Calgary for the Spring Conference at Prairie again. Am I running ahead of the Lord? I don't want to do that, or have I become over confident, and let down on my 'pressing on'? Am I feeling that I have 'arrived'? I don't think so. The one thing I do know, is that God is not the Author of confusion, and that He who has begun a good work in us will perfect it, or bring it to full completion. He is leading, He is the Light of the world, and He has told us that if we follow Him, we will not walk in darkness, but will have the light of life.

"Oh, light my way, dear Lord, that I might be obedient!"

April 7, 1986

I called Al Mount this morning, and he told me that the council had discussed the situation in Haiti, and decided that I should not go yet. I was to wait and go to the program at the Master's College first, and then go to Haiti for three months, which will put me into June after the program; so I changed my last day of work, and needless to say, they were glad since we are so short on nights right now. I did ask for vacation time so I could go to Prairie, and they gave it to me.

Last Wednesday, just before I went to bed to take my 'night nap' before going to work all night, I got a phone call from Erik Bjorn at Prairie. He and his family are going to have me stay with them, and they will pick me up at the airport. I hope they don't feel they owe me something for sending John's tapes to them this last year, and I'm concerned over how they will get them when I go to Haiti? I've been trying to build up his library, but there are so many tapes!

The Lord had also given me the privilege of buying John's study guides for a fellow who had stopped by the tape library window one Sunday morning about two months ago. He was rather scruffy looking, and his hair was unkempt and long. In the course of conversation, he said he'd like to have some of John's books. He told me he was out of work, and living in his van.

I said that if it wouldn't offend him, I would be glad to get some of them for him, and he accepted. Every week he was back to show me how he had studied them, and they were all underlined, and marked up with his notes. Then, he'd pick up another five or six and leave. About the third week, he told me how his view was changing on the security of the believer, and he had cut his hair. Then, Easter Sunday, a member of Grace Church, who is an L.A. detective, stopped by the tape shack, and pulled me aside. He told me that the church had decided not to help this man anymore, since he was not even trying to get a job, and had refused to do any of the jobs available at the church. I told him, "If that was the elder's decision, I will go along with that, and respect their decision."

When I told the fellow of their decision, he immediately became rather hostile, especially against policeman, though I had not said who had told me. But, then as we talked, he calmed down some and left.

I was disappointed when he didn't show up the next Sunday. I was hoping he would tell me that he had gotten a job. Instead, he told me that there were only two people at Grace Church that he would accept correction from, – me and John MacArthur! That was really putting me in great company!

I told him it was done in love, and that I could no longer buy books for him. I've been praying for him, – his attitude needs some serious changing. He was upset because he was being told to go to work, when he was busy studying God's Word! I tried to tell him that there are many – me included – who'd love to spend every day in the Word, but that we had to work to eat, and to be able to help others! Maybe he will show up again; I'll keep praying for him anyway.

I forgot an added blessing about going to Prairie. John is going to be the speaker at the graduation, and will be having his noon meal at Erik Bjorn's house, and so will I! Canada seems like a long way to go to have dinner with your Pastor, but I'm really excited. With such a large congregation as Grace Church, it's nearly impossible to ever get to talk to John, and I'm sure he will be surprised when he sees the same face that peers up at him from the fifth row on Sundays, across the table from him in Canada!

April 14, 1986

Lord willing, I'll leave early tomorrow morning for Prairie. My friend, Susan, that I met last year at Prairie, called this morning, and she has decided to come to the Conference too! Great!

Today, the U.S. attacked Lybia. What comfort, and how calming, to know that the One who is in control of all of it, is the very same One who holds my life in the hollow of His nail scarred hands. It's sad to see people fret and fume over world events. God has a plan, and no one, not Reagan, not Khadaffi, nor the Russians, is able to change anything. He is still the Sovereign Lord of all He has created! Amen!

April 20, 1986 At Prairie

It's been a good week here at Prairie. What fault there has been I'm sure lies within me, and not with anything external. I enjoyed my visit with the Bjorn's, and appreciated their generous hospitality. The anticipated noon meal with John and his wife, Patricia, was, as Erik's wife put it – awesome! They are such a truly gracious couple! John's messages have been so good, and so well received, but they have let him have so little time! What a waste of an opportunity to sit under one of God's choice teachers in not letting him speak as often as he would.

Major Thomas, another speaker, is growing old, with the smacking mouth, and trembling knees, but his messages were good. He truly loves the Lord, but there's only one John.

May 24, 1986

Last night was my last night at work. It's such a thrill and a joy to see God's hand moving so obviously in my life.

On Wednesday night, I took some counted cross stitch to work with me, but forgot the material to do it on, so I couldn't do any of it. So – because I was left with nothing to do, except work, I went down to the ER to see if the doctor there would write a prescription for chloroquin, (a prophylactic for malaria) which he did, and Otto in the pharmacy ordered it for me. Then I asked if I could get a tetanus shot as well, and they obliged. How good the Lord is! I'm all ready to go. I got the free hepatitis shots already, and now, getting this done two days before I'm no longer an employee is really helpful. I had no plan to do this, it just all fell into place at just the right time.

Then, though I was given the choice, I had already said, "On this my last night here, Lord, please put me where You want me." So, I was back in the Preemie Room. I wondered who the Lord would give me an opportunity to talk to, and it was Chutima, whose name means 'Light in a dark place.' She is a Buddhist from Thailand, but is open to talking about spiritual things. We had an hour or more when neither of us had a chore to do, a miracle in itself with six babies to feed, and so we talked. The problem was, she doesn't feel she is a sinner, therefore, she has no need. How sad to be so blinded to the truth. She hasn't worked at Northridge in two months, and only works there one night a week – on my last night. I must remember to pray for her.

Then, another girl, who hasn't worked here for several months either, and though I had no opportunity to talk to her, she told me her brother was working downstairs, and I know him as a strong Christian, while his family is Buddhist. I asked her to tell him to come up and see me when he could. He has been such a blessing to me. Having found the Lord, (the Lord found him) all by himself, he has grown in the Lord so beautifully, and is a real joy! When we are together, the only thing we talk about is the Lord and His truth, and we both go away filled with the joy of the Lord. I love him as my 'little Japanese brother' in Christ. I really expect the Lord will use him in wonderful ways for His glory!

Now, as the Lord closes one door, and opens another – how wonderful to wait upon Him, trust in Him, and lean upon Him for all my needs. My Father owns the cattle on a thousand hills, and I know He cares for me. Yet, in all my reading and listening, I keep hearing these words over and over - suffering, persecution, trials, testing, and I wonder what the Lord is telling me, and what might be in store for me? I know that these things are all part of being a Christian, and we shouldn't be surprised when they come.

Haiti is in such an unstable state right now, and the Communists are just waiting for the right moment to try to take over. I wonder if I will be caught up in some kind of political trouble there? I've talked to the Lord about it, and I can honestly say that 'I count not my life as dear unto myself, and to depart and be with Christ is far better.' Whatever will glorify Him – life or death – it really doesn't matter. " To me to live is Christ, and to die is gain." Philippians 1:21 KJV Praise the Lord!

June 5, 1986 Father's Day

My little Daddy has been with the Lord for nearly four years now, and what joy it must be for him to always behold the face of his Lord Jesus!

I just felt that I must write in this, as time is passing. My three weeks of Missionary Internship and Language Orientation, have come and gone. Some of it was interesting, some was fun, and some was painful. Some of it exposed my shortcomings far too clearly, and I'm not too pleased with what I saw about myself. Most of the other participants were very young (20's) and I really didn't have much in common with them, outside of Christ. It made it difficult for me to enter in and participate, as I felt they were uncomfortable with me. I always seem to be the odd man. (Either that or I am really paranoid.)

They are wonderful, sweet young people, and I know the Lord will use them.

Language Orientation brought another Prairie grad into my life. He was the instructor, and I discovered that he and Al Mount were in my husband, Andy's class at Prairie way back in the 1950's. Amazing!

Well, I am almost at the stepping off place. Kathy, my daughter, is coming tomorrow, and we'll go to Tonopah to visit the boys. After that, I just don't know.

I wonder if I will see John again before I leave. He will be gone for several weeks, and I may leave before he gets back. I will miss Grace Church sorely! Yet, I can't keep feasting in the green pasture there, but I must begin to give back now.

All I could think of was Psalm 44:11 and 22 "Thou hast given us like sheep, appointed for meat; and hast scattered us among the heathen.. . . . Yea, for Thy sake are we killed all the day long; we are counted as sheep for the slaughter." KJV

Sheep are well fed before they are killed, and I have been feasting at a spiritual smorgasbord here at Grace. Now, I am so fat, and ready for whatever God has for me.

My hearts desires are:
1. That God will confirm or deny my call to Haiti while I am there.
2. That I will be sensitive to the people and their needs.
3. That God will give me a genuine love for the people of Haiti, and for those I will be working with there.
4. That God will give me a friend there to be accountable to.
5. That He will constantly show me how to give myself away, and to pour out my life for Him.

I seem to be so superficial, and I don't know how to give of myself. I can give things, and money, oh yes, but the real inner me – no. I pray that He will do a real work in me, however painful it may be – that I might be transparent, and able to love as He loves.

June 30, 1986

Last day of June! What a great and loving God our God is. Truly He is a loving Father who loves to give good gifts to His children!

Dr. Benson called me this morning to tell me that Agape Flights is filled, and they can't take me, so I'll have to fly with MAF, Mission Aviation Fellowship, my favorite airline, and the one I wanted to go on! Also, not on the eighteenth of July, but on the twenty-second. The Lord knew that I really wanted to stay and be here for this Sunday at Grace. John will bring both morning and evening messages, and I was so wishing that I could just put off going for those few days, but I knew I had to go when I was told to. Isn't it marvelous the way God worked it out for me?! I'll be here for Sunday, the twentieth, I'll leave for Florida on the twenty-first, and leave for Haiti on the twenty-second. It was perfect planning. What a wonderful surprise gift from my gracious and loving Lord! His word is true, and His promises are sure. "Delight thyself in the Lord, and He shall give thee the desires of thine heart. Commit thy way unto the Lord; trust also in Him, and He shall bring it to pass."

Psalm 37: 4 and 5 KJV

He's also shown me how I can go from Port-au- Prince to Cap-Haitien very easily without anyone having to take me – MAF flies between the two cities for $25.00. Marvelous! No problem! I'll be able to go see Al Warren and his wife – Praise the Lord!

Monnie Brewer is feeling even more unsure about Medical Ambassadors for me, and has said he doesn't feel I should go to their board meeting on the tenth, as he feels that is like making a commitment for me. I don't know what to tell Dr. Benson since I already wrote to tell him I would come. He was very happy, and I was glad to be able to do something to please him, but now, I'll just have to wait and see what the Lord will do, and He will do something, I know. He is so good to me, and I don't deserve anything from Him.

July 13, 1986

Well, I wrote Dr. Benson a letter and explained to him why I wasn't coming to the board meeting, and last Monday, I took it to Monnie to read before I mailed it, and he said it was OK. I found out tonight that Monnie also wrote to Dr. Benson, and told him that they had not wanted me to go. They have been so supportive of me all along the way, but tonight really topped it off. What a great and wonderful God we serve and love.

This is what Grace Church did tonight that really topped it off. They handed me a check for one thousand dollars!! I am still stunned. I know I don't deserve it, but then the Lord doesn't give us gifts because we deserve them, but for us to use them to bring Him glory. How gracious of Him, He is ever the God of grace!

I told Monnie, I really didn't need that much, but he said the board had decided on that amount, and that I should just put it away. Do you think God can't supply your needs? Try Him! He has supplied mine before I even knew I had the need. Amen!

"How can I say thanks for the things You have done for me, Things so undeserved, yet You've given to show Your love for me. The voices of a million angels could not express my gratitude. All that I am, or ever hope to be, I owe it all to You!"

Written by Andre Crouch

July 18, 1986

I didn't think I needed that money, but today, when I bought my Traveler's Checks, I found I really did. God KNEW I did, so He made sure that I had what I needed. Praise our faithful Heavenly Father, who takes SUCH GOOD care of His own.

July 19, 1986

I've been reading L.E. Maxwell's little book called, "World Missions: Total War"

It's an excellent book, one I will recommend for the Missions Preparation list of books for Stage I. But, what I wanted to include here – my next to last night before I leave for Haiti – is this sentence:

"There is time for you, latecomer though you be, to win a battle before your sun goes down."

Amen! I hope it's a great and glorious battle to the death – death of self, pride, selfishness, or even physical death – it matters not, so long as the battle is won for Christ!

In Haiti

July 21, 1986

I took the Fly-A-Way bus from the valley to the airport to catch the 11am Delta flight to Fort Lauderdale, Florida. The plane was about forty-five minutes late leaving L.A. Airport, so it arrived in Florida late, but the van from Howard Johnson's was still there waiting for me. It's very warm and humid here in Florida, not at all like California.

I have a very nice room with a shower, though I decided to take a shower, and wash my hair in the morning. It's difficult to go to sleep due to the time change, but I need to get up by 4:30 in the morning, to be ready by 5:45 to leave for the Missionary Flights hanger.

July 22, 1986

I was up at 4:30am to shower and wash my hair. I want to have a bit of breakfast so I can take my malaria prophylaxis, chloriquin. To my dismay, the shower didn't work, so I got down on my hands and knees to bathe and wash my hair under the spout on the tub. Then, I ran over to Denny's across the street, and got a bite to eat. Then, I ran back across the street to my room, got my bags, and the van took me to the Missionary Flights hanger, where I waited for about an hour.

At a little before 7am, we took off for Cap-Haitien, and the expression, 'the plane lumbered down the runway' was so true! We flew in a 1943 vintage DC-3, with a center aisle that slanted up when we boarded. We, all four passengers, were asked to sit forward to help balance the cargo. We flew to Georgetown in the Bahamas, and refueled there, which took about fifteen minutes, and then we were back in the air.

We arrived in Cap-Haitien about noon. When I got to the open door of the plane to get out, I felt like someone had slapped a hot rag that smelled like garbage in my face.

It was very hot and humid, and the garbage lining the streets was responsible for the aroma. The weather was just what I had anticipated; temperature in the eighty to ninety degree range, and a humidity of seventy to eighty percent. Very hot and sticky!

The airport is very small, and the customs officials just waved me through, without even opening my bags. (Sure different than Saudi Arabia, where they paw through everything.)

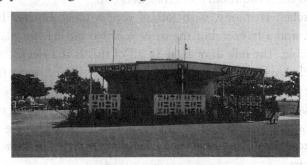

The airport in Cap-Haitien

Flo, who will be my room mate, arrived to collect me, and we drove (if you want to call it that) to the house. Flo is a real 'no nonsense' older nurse, whom the Lord called to Haiti when she was sixty years old. She is nearly deaf, and wears hearing aids in both ears. A headband is also worn so the sweat won't ruin her hearing aids.

It was a real 'white knuckle' ride to the house, and I remember asking the Lord, *"Oh, Lord, did you call me here to die, before I even get started?"*

Another wonderful surprise – it was a beautiful house – rather like a California mission style, with lots of iron work on the door, windows, and porch railings. There was a heavy wooden door, and a two color tile floor inside, which carried out to the nice front porch as well. All of the windows had iron grillwork, and screens, which surprised me. The living room, which went all the way across the front of the house, was furnished with a pretty light wood corner cupboard, a futon, Flo's recliner, her piano, and several Haitian chairs, with cane seats, plus there was a very nice ceiling fan with three lights.

The windows all have shutters that fold inward, but are kept open most of the time, as is the front door. The iron grill door is closed and locked, to discourage people from just walking in unannounced.

There are three bedrooms, and two bathrooms. There are three of us here right now; Flo, and a young girl named Susie, who has just graduated from Nursing School. Now I am added to the mix. Flo has the very back bedroom, and it has a private bathroom with a bathtub, and a shower. Susie and I will share the other bathroom, which has a shower, plus, it also has the washer and dryer. We each have a very nice bedroom, with a twin bed each. The bedrooms each have a window over the head of the bed, with a screen on it. Every once in awhile a soft cool breeze blows over you, and it feels SO good! Some clever person has put screen doors on each bedroom, which keeps the mosquitoes and tarantulas out!

The kitchen is roomy, with lots of nice wood cabinets. There is a refrigerator, and a freezer, but the stove is a two burner hot plate sitting on a long table. The one draw-back in all of this is the electricity, which is very unreliable, and is known to go off frequently, and sometimes stays off for long periods of time.

Water is another problem. Our water comes from a spring up on the mountain behind us, through a long pipe to our cistern, where it is then pumped into the house by - electricity. Frequent power surges wreak havoc on the motors.

The people get their water from public faucets along the highway, and some even take their bath there.

Flo has hired several men to work around the house, cleaning the car, watering the plants, washing off the front porch, etc. We also have a housekeeper, Ma'Louie, who comes at 12:30pm, washes dishes, hangs out the clothes that have been washed, irons them, cleans the house, and cooks our dinner, and then goes home at 5pm. She is a very sweet quiet lady whose husband works in the clinic. We also have a night watchman who sits all night on the porch with his big machete.

Poor missionaries indeed! This is FAR better than I've ever had it, anywhere!

What I've seen so far is very nice, especially when I was expecting, I didn't know what. I was SO hot, sticky, and miserable the day I arrived, that I wondered how long I would be able to stand it, but when I see how the people live, I feel extremely thankful!

I am confused about a lot of things, but I'm sure it will all straighten out in time. Flo is very hard of hearing, so it's difficult to ask her questions, but Susie has proven to be a gold-mine of information, and she's only been here for six weeks. She has picked up a lot of the Creole language, and has great fun trying to talk to everyone.

We had a Bible study here my first night, so I met a few more folks who are missionaries here. There were twelve here, and the fellow who gave the Bible study was charismatic, and believes that any sickness is from the devil, and we should not allow it. I felt that he didn't understand James 1:2 very well, " My brethren, count it all joy when you fall into various trials,. . ." We are to expect all kinds of trials, including sickness, as these help us to grow and trust God with everything. We can't stop the devil, he is much more powerful than we are, but God is able, and He will take care of our foe. Their situation is especially sad, because his wife is in a wheel chair, and they feel that, if they had enough faith, she would walk again.

When the Bible study was over, I took a lovely cool shower, and it felt wonderful! I can't believe I'm really here, Praise the Lord!

July 23, 1986

Today was my first Clinic day; got up early, and walked to the clinic. It's about a half mile away, at Providence Orphanage. There were people waiting with lots of kids. I met quite a few workers, some Haitian, and some American; we had a short devotional time, and then went out and gave out cards with numbers on them. As you walk down the line of waiting people, you try to assess who is the sickest, by feeling foreheads. The hottest get seen first. This is their way of doing a triage.

One of the workers weighs the kids, and another checks their ears, and asks the mom what the symptoms are. She then sends them to another of the workers who asks more questions, and tries to diagnosis what the problem is. She then writes a prescription, and sends them to the 'piki' (shot) room for a shot of antibiotic, or some oral re-hydration, and then to the clinic pharmacy where they receive their medicine with instructions how to take it, or give it.

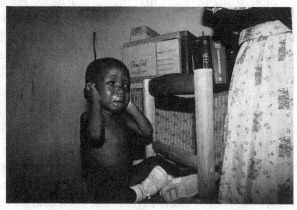

A child in our clinic

A few of the kids were really sick. One of them was a two year old, whose mother had gotten sick, and the grand-mother was caring for the child. This child was very emaciated, and her skin was dry, cracking, and peeling. Her lips were cracked, and she was very weak, and could hardly cry. Several small babies looked almost comatose.

I sat with one of the American women, who was diagnosing, but she seemed rather unsure at times, and I can understand why. So many sicknesses here present with similar symptoms, and without any x-ray or lab tests, all you can do sometimes, is make an educated guess, and hope you're right. We were there until 2:30, and saw about sixty kids.

One little boy had only a shirt on, and no pants; several of the little girls wore dresses, but had no panties. Some were way over dressed, even though they had high fevers, and even the small babies had sweaters and booties on – in this heat! I guess it's a status symbol. Most of the babies had no diaper, only a towel under them.

It was very obvious which babies were breast fed, and which were bottle fed. The breast fed babies were plump and quite healthy looking, with good growth. The bottle fed babies were very skinny, and were not thriving or growing normally. The bottle is also a status symbol here unfortunately. They have a big poster hanging on the wall that someone has made; it's a picture of a big baby bottle with a shriveled, very skinny baby inside. Across the top it says, 'The Bottle is Death' in Créole. Pretty impressive, I thought.

One little boy, about two years old, had little pig-tails all over his head, like a girl. He wasn't talking yet, and they don't cut a boy's hair here until he talks, or he will never talk, so they believe.

Today hasn't seemed quite so hot to me. There was some cloud cover, and a nice breeze. (Still not Hawaii, though!) After dinner, Susie and I took a long walk, and took our cameras along. We saw a lot, and learned quite a bit as well.

I learned that there ARE some trees here. I had read that they had cut them all down. Some of the trees are very big, and the mountains behind the house seem very big, and they are green with mist covering the tops. I've seen mango, breadfruit, and banana trees here so far, and I've seen corn growing. I've also seen a lot of indescribable places, with people actually living in them. Several of the people asked for money, probably because I was a new white face.

There were many 'tap-taps', which are usually small pick-up trucks with a camper shell. They are the Haitian public transportation, and are called 'tap-taps' because when you want to get off, you tap, (bang loudly) with your hand on the side of the truck or bus, so the driver will stop and let you off.

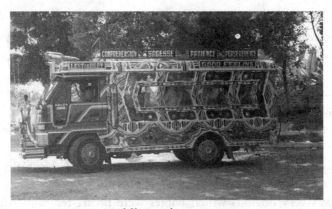

Middle sized tap-tap

They are painted with all kinds of decorations, and usually have a religious inscription across the front, sort of like a prayer. This is to protect everyone from accidents, which happen often. Larger, big busses were screaming along, laying on the horn every so often. The 'tap-taps are the local bus, and the big busses, called camions, are the express between the cities. It costs 1 goud, or twenty cents to ride the tap-tap, and this is when you experience real Haitian 'togetherness'. People are packed in like sardines, and where there is a shortage of soap and water, it's a real sensory experience in this hot and humid country!

There are lots of bicycles, scooters, some motorcycles, and cars. Also, lots of pitiful little donkeys, with beautiful saddles made from some kind of plant leaf, probably banana. There are cows, goats, chickens, and dogs everywhere. ALL of them are skinny, with their ribs showing; a few cats, but they get eaten. However, Flo has a very fat cat named Nikki, and it's a wonder she hasn't been eaten yet.

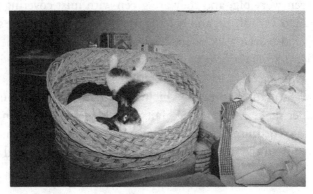

Flo's cat, Nikki

Driving here reminds me of those game machines where you put a quarter in the slot, and as you move the steering wheel people, animals, and other cars jump out in your path, and the challenge is to NOT hit them. That's what driving in Haiti is like. It's a choreographed disaster waiting to happen! Plus, if you do hit someone, you are then liable for everything they need, and if you should accidentally kill someone, the people who witness it will probably kill you, so what people do – is just keep on driving.

The women walk, carrying their bundles on their heads effortlessly, and the little kids, 'ti-mouns' all point at us and yell, "Blanc, blanc", which means "white, white!"

July 24, 1986

It's a day of rest today, with no clinics. I moved a nice big table into my room, so now I have a desk for my tapes, radio, and books. It's a bit large, but it's nice to have my own spot.

This evening, Susie and I went for a walk in the other direction from last night, and we saw lots more interesting things. It's fun to walk with her, as she just chats with everyone, and laughs with them.

One of the things we saw tonight on our walk was a group of men playing a game of dominoes. They hold them in their hands and slap them down on a table, and you can always tell who's losing, because he will have clothes-pins on his face! One poor fellow must have been a real loser, as he had them pinching both his cheeks from his ears to his chin. He looked so funny that Suzy asked if she could take a picture, but he was so humiliated that he said "No!" while all his fellow players were yelling, "Yes! Yes!"

Last night there was a lot more traffic than there has been, and it was due to a fête, or celebration, in a town called Plaine du Nord. It was a 'mud bath' party, and everybody was going. It is a mud baptism connected with voodoo, and people come from many different countries in the world to attend. In fact, Plaine du Nord is called the voodoo capital of the world. Our next door neighbor, Sandy went, just to see what it was all about, and some woman who was in the mud hole tried to pull him in. He came home with mud all over his clothes and a rather frightened look on his face.

There was laughing and singing, and drums all night long. I had a hard time going to sleep.

July 25, 1986

We were all up early this morning, loading up Flo's Daihatsu, four-wheel- drive Rocky, with medicine and water. We picked up two American missionaries, Kathy and Alice, and a Haitian fellow named Ronnie, and off we went to a village in the mountains called San Raphael.

It was a long drive, about an hour and a half, and we ran out of paved roads, and hit rough, rocky roads that wound up and up, and over streams with no bridges. I was so thankful for the air-conditioning in the car, so we could keep the windows up, otherwise, we'd have been covered with dust. We passed lots of people, thatched huts, cows, goats, chickens, donkeys, horses, and little naked kids everywhere!

There are lots of trees in this area! There are banana, mango, breadfruit, papaya, coconut, and lots of other trees of different kinds that I don't recognize. On the way up the mountain, we had a great view of 'The Citadel', which is a huge fortress-castle, built by Henri Christophe, one of Haiti's many dictator kings. It is an empty, tourist attraction now, and they say it is a difficult climb to get to it.

When we finally arrived at the village, the people were all there, waiting for us. The clinic was to be held in the church there, with it's lime washed mud walls, and dirt floor. Some sick folks were lying on a mat on the floor. We laid out the medicines on a table, gave out our numbers, and tried to gain some order from the chaos. We had a corner screened off with two sheets, and four of us sat in there, two of us per patient. We called out, "Number one", and away we went.

I can't believe it, I've been here two days, and now I am a 'Doctor'. I have to diagnose, and prescribe medicines for adults; some with problems I've never even heard of before! Once in awhile, I think, maybe I've managed to give something that will help the person. At least the Aspirin and Tylenol might help with the fevers, and the aches and pains of the old ones. There was only one patient that I felt I might be qualified to treat, and that was a tiny baby, two months old, but it couldn't have weighed five pounds at most. It was very pale and listless, with too many clothes on.

It was a pretty, sweet little thing, but its mama said that it wouldn't eat. She fed it twice a day, but she didn't tell me what she fed it. I asked for a

85

bottle of formula, with a preemie nipple on it, and I tried to feed the baby. It gagged a little, but I persisted, and it finally took about three fourths of a cc., which isn't even one ounce. I hated to give it up. I wanted to keep it and feed it, but we tried to tell the mom how to do it. I hope she's able to keep it alive. It would have been in the NICU at home, with IV's, and every two hour feedings, or hyperalimentation solution, via IV. So sad, so many babies die here just like this of dehydration and malnutrition.

Then I treated old folks with numerous aches and pains, probably from the very hard lives they have lived, and they are now in their fifties and sixties, which is pretty old here. There were a couple of cases of venereal diseases, but I have no idea which, though probably syphilis. Flo delights in giving them a whopping shot of painfully thick penicillin.

Several people were so sick they couldn't walk without help. One lady was delirious, and had a large lump on the side of her head, and one little girl was just burning up with fever. Some of these really sick ones – with lumps here and there, or shortness of breath, etc. – we sent to the mission Doctor in another town, with a note for him, telling him that we had sent them. All we could do was treat symptoms.

I sat there thinking, how wonderful it would have been, if like in those Bible towns where Jesus went, and healed all their diseases, we could have just spoken a word and they would have been healed. I wished that He could have been there in the flesh with us, to touch, and heal all of these people. He wouldn't even have to ask what their symptoms were, He'd already know, and it wouldn't matter anyway, as all it would take would be a word, or touch from the Master. How His tender heart must weep with ours, at this sad product of sin called disease.

I feel so inadequate, and yet they look to me as if I could make all of their pain and misery, go away. *"Oh, Lord, if only I could!"*

And then, after you prescribe Antacid, Aspirin, and vitamins, they are so grateful, and tell you 'thank you', as though you had given them the world.

Some of the old folks told me they had 'gaz,' and they would pat their head, their stomach, their knees, or their arms and legs. I could only call it 'traveling gas,' and figured it had to be pain they were trying to describe to me. One man complained of 'wind in his ears' and some told me that their hands or legs were 'dead', yet they were able to move them. How does one treat 'wind in the ears' or 'dead limbs'? I really wish I knew! We started about 10:30am, and finished about 3:30pm, without a break of any kind. My problem was my ears. They really started to hurt from my stethoscope after a couple of hours, but the people don't feel that you have really examined them if you haven't listened to their heart and chest, and taken their blood pressure. One blood pressure I took was 200/140. Poor old lady probably won't be around much longer with a blood pressure like that. All we can give them is a diuretic, but it frequently works quite well. When the clinic was over, Pastor Livingston, who is blind, said we must come and eat, as his wife had prepared a real feast for us. They had given her money the week before to buy what she needed for the meal.

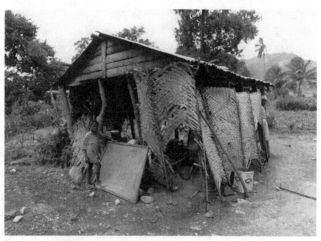

The kitchen where our meal was cooked

We had a spicy goat meat stew, which was very tasty, but very spicy, and my mouth burned all the way back down the mountain! She also made rice with a tasty black bean sauce, a salad, potatoes, and carrots. It was very good, and it was all cooked outside on a charcoal fire. We ate in the dining room of their house, which has mud walls, dirt floor, and four rooms for eight people. I noticed a spider skeleton hanging on the wall, sort of like some kind of macabre décor.

We had to use an outhouse, which was also decorated with spider skeleton décor, but I was happy that we didn't have to use a bush, because everyone isn't fortunate enough to have an outhouse, and it seems that there is always someone, already behind every bush.

Well, after we ate, we all piled back into the Rocky, and drove back down the mountain. We got back home about 5:30pm, which made for a good long day, but it was so interesting, and it went by very quickly.

Pastor Livingston has several children, but, one, a little boy eight years old, is showing the same symptoms in his eyes as his father had, before he went blind, and when Flo goes back to the States, she wants to take him with her so he can be evaluated by doctors there. His name is Dieu-donnez, which means 'God given'.

July 26, 1986

I did a lot of errands today, and this evening Susie and I went to Kathy and Alice's house which is several miles down the road. They are working with a Haitian pastor who has built a compound, consisting of a big church, a clinic where he uses his own plant medicines, which he makes himself. There is also an orphanage, a school, and a house where Kathy and Alice live. Susie rounded up about twenty-five of the orphans, sat them up on some planks of wood across some saw-horses, got out her guitar, and they had a 'sing.' Boy, do they love to sing – in Créole and in English! They really enjoyed it.

One little four year old girl named Magdala, began getting sleepier and sleepier, until, finally, she began to nod, and her eyes began to close. I was afraid she would fall off the plank, so I picked her up, sat her on my lap where she could lean against me, and she just snored away, while everyone else sang.

Alice then brought out a cake she'd made, but which had fallen in the middle. She'd iced it anyway; cut it up into small pieces and gave it to the kids.

July 27, 1986

We got up and went to church at É.B.A.C.(Église Baptiste Armé du Christ) or the Baptist Church Army of Christ compound where Kathy and Alice live; the two who had gone with us to the clinic yesterday.

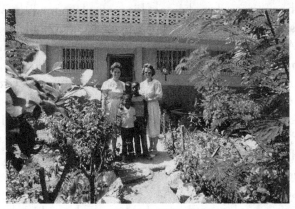

Kathy and Alice standing in front of their house with three of the orphans

It was a special day for the churches here, called Harvest Festival, and there were six Baptist churches participating, with the six pastors there. The church was a large cement block building, built so the air could flow through the walls. It also had five large ceiling fans, but it was still hot!. The church was all festooned with – toilet paper of different colors, all draped in long chains every where! There were three choirs, and a group of five girls who sang together. It was very nice, and the music was wonderful! The church even has a real organ that Kathy plays, but she told me that the pedals for the bass don't work anymore because the rats ate the felt off of them. She said that the rats used to run out on her feet when she'd begin to play!

The sermon was good, I guess, because I couldn't understand it. I enjoyed just watching everyone.

One little toddler kept getting away from his mom, and wandering all over. His older sister caught him several times, but in another few minutes, he'd be wandering again, with his thumb in his mouth. During the sermon, about every five minutes, a rooster would loudly crow. It sounded like it was right in the room – and it might have been.

After church, we went to the Hotel Mont Jolie, and it was like being in another world. It's a very nice tourist hotel, with a beautiful view of the ocean and bay, a nice swimming pool, and tables outside where we could sit and eat. We had a nice lunch, and I had an 'omelette créole', which was very tasty. Susie and Flo even had ice cream for dessert.

This evening, we went to the English Church in the town, where most of the missionaries go. A young man gave an inspiring testimony.

July 28, 1986

Clinic again today at Providence Orphanage, and again, I sat with a more experienced worker, while she diagnosed little 'ti- moun', which is children in Créole.

It literally is 'little men', but means both girls and boys, or children.

There were several very sick kids again. They look like they feel absolutely miserable, and I'm sure most of them do.

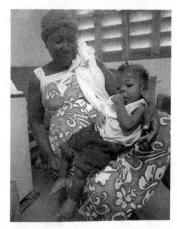

A child in our clinic probably suffering from Kwashiorkor protein deficiency

One little boy was there with his father who has TB and is blind from a brain tumor which is slowly killing him; so we gave the dad his TB medicine and some Tylenol with codeine for his pain. His little boy, Jason was also sick, but was leading his father around with a stick held between them. So sad! My heart breaks over the physical suffering of some of these people.

One young mother had quit nursing her six month old baby, who was sick and so skinny. She had quit because she was pregnant again, and they believe that it will hurt or kill the second child if they continue to nurse the first, so they quit, and frequently it's the first child who dies of malnutrition instead.

There is a mission hospital a few miles up the road in a town called Limbé where there are several Christian doctors, and we sent some of the sickest kids to them. We saw about eighty kids, and went from 7:30am to 2:30 pm without a break.

After lunch, Susie, Ronnie our translator, and I went to the Iron Market in Cap-Haitien. It's always good to have Ronnie along as he speaks excellent English, and can translate for us.

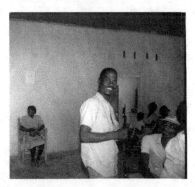

Ronnie, our translator and friend

The Iron Market defies description! It was the most filthy, smelly, place – worse than the Bahta in Riyadh, Saudi Arabia, and that was BAD!

With Ronnie's help, we bought twelve nice tomatoes for one dollar, six very small heads of lettuce for a dollar and eighty cents, and two avocados for twenty cents. They all have to go in the Clorox dip before we eat them. Susie bought two little dresses for two dollars and fifty cents each, and I bought eight pair of little girl's panties, for fifty cents a pair. They are for some of the little girls at the orphanage. Then we went to the French bakery, and bought cookies and some croissants.

After dinner, Susie and I went for another walk. We were looking for a young mom with a sick baby. We had told her to bring the baby to the clinic, but we had told her the wrong day in Créole. We found her – she lives in one of the huts along the street, and we put some erythromycin eye ointment in the baby's eyes. When we had seen it in the clinic a couple of days ago, only its eyes were infected, now it also has a runny nose and diarrhea. We told her to bring the baby to the clinic on Wednesday, so we can see how it is doing.

A man riding a scooter, and pulling a small two wheeled trailer, stopped and ever so politely, in the grandest English, said he was there to help us "in any way I can!" He was so nice, but we never saw him again.

On our way back home, a very poor old lady was telling us how sick she was, and could she please have some money? She didn't even have any shoes on, poor pitiful old soul. I feel so guilty that I have SO much, and they all have SO little, or nothing!

July 29, 1986

"He that hath pity upon the poor lendeth unto the Lord, and that which he hath given, will He pay him again."

Proverbs 19:17 KJV

The Living Bible says it this way, "When you help the poor, you are lending to the Lord – and He pays wonderful interest on your loan!"

Proverbs 19:17

What a great verse for Haiti! There are so many poor – the poorest of the poor. I want to give them everything I have, but as soon as you do, they become yours forever, and there will be ten more just as desperate as the first one, at your door. *Oh, Dear Lord, what do you do?* It breaks my heart to say 'no' to a wrinkled, toothless face, with white fuzz for hair, calloused old feet with no shoes, and rags where clothes should be.

To be torn in two directions is so painful, but I never want to become hardened to the pitiful plight of these precious people. Human beings, who have been reduced to living like animals by the cruelest taskmaster there is – Satan himself.

Haiti is an example of what Satan will give you if you follow him – sickness, poverty, filth, hunger, and pain, and finally, death and Hell. The Haitians dedicate their land to Satan every year, and then wonder why they have to live like they do. I can't imagine having to live in such an abject, desperate state your whole life on this earth, and then, when you die – Hell awaits.

Then, because they are so poor, they lie, cheat, and steal. I can't really blame them for trying to get something, when they have nothing, and for most people here, there is absolutely no way to earn anything, as there is no work available. They are willing to work, long and hard, but there are so few jobs for so many people. That is one reason Flo hires helpers for the house; it gives us more time, and it helps them earn money, which then helps their families, and gives them some self respect. They remain amazingly sweet considering what they have been reduced to in life. I have watched them being cruel to their animals, which I really hate to see, but when you have been reduced to living like an animal, yourself, it must be pretty hard to care about their suffering.

July 30, 1986

We saw about sixty-five kids today in the clinic, and again, some very sick ones. One baby had about six big bumps all over his head, and I don't know what they were.(The only other baby I have seen with lumps like this was a baby in the hospital in Saudi Arabia, and it was diagnosed as cancer.)

There were rashes, coughs, runny noses, dirt, non-stop crying, and sticky heat.

The clinic is really a disaster area as far as organization of supplies. Flo knows where things are, but I can never find what I am looking for. There are boxes everywhere, and each one has an assortment of things in it.

The clinic will be closing for good soon, per Dr. Benson's order, as he feels that the pastor at the orphanage is not doing his share, and that his life is not what it should be.

Flo feels that the best way is to teach some, and then let them go and teach their own villages. I feel that this is probably the best way to care for them, because with some knowledge, they can prevent a lot of the sickness we see now. So many of their problems are the result of poor hygiene, compounded by malnutrition, because no one has taught them anything about germs and hygiene.

They don't know the simplest things, like boiling river water before making baby formula which, alone could save numberless babies, but they have no idea.

I am still confused about how all of the clinics and people fit together. I still don't know who is working for whom, or for which organization. No one volunteers much information, or bothers to introduce different people who show up from time to time.

It's very, very hot and sticky, and I seem to have a deep cough which is hanging on from the cold I had before I came. Also, we have gotten another room-mate, an R.N. named Anne, who has been here before.

August 1, 1986

We spent yesterday getting ready to go to Port-au- Prince. We left this morning about 10am, stopped to pick up Kathy and Alice, and we were off. It was a four hour, thrill-a-minute ride, dodging people, goats, cattle, chickens, dogs, tap-taps and trucks. Then there are the pot-holes! You dodge one, only to fall into two more.

This is the only road from Cap-Haitien in the north, and Port-au-Prince in the south. It is only a two lane road which winds over very high mountains, with spectacular views of more mountains in the distance. Thatched roof huts, waterfalls, trees and rivers are everywhere. No matter how far away from a village or town you get, there are always people along the roadside, walking somewhere, with something. The women carry huge loads on their heads, and with no effort at all, they swing along down the road with wide baskets filled with produce or charcoal, and sometimes it's a big pot of water. If I tried to do that, there would be an empty pot by the time I got it home!

We finally arrived in Port-au-Prince, and went to the home of a Mennonite couple who run a guest house there. They have nine year old twin girls, Rachel and Rhoda, who have long blond braids. It was a very nice house, but our room was on the front, where it was unbelievably noisy.

August 2, 1986

We got up and had breakfast, and then we made "Rocky" climb another hill, all the way up to 4,000 feet to the Baptist Haiti Mission. There is a church, a small hospital, an outlet store, and a cafeteria style restaurant with a fabulous view of terraced hillsides growing all kinds of seedling trees, flowers, and vegetables, which they sell. The outlet store has some pretty hand embroidered clothing, plus carved wooden objects, a few books, and other trinkets of all kinds. I bought some clothes, since I love anything embroidered. Then, we ate lunch in their restaurant, and it was very good.

Baptist Haiti Mission began as a sample farm for the mountain people, and it's grown into a big complex, which now includes cabins for other missionaries to stay in for vacations, or like we did, just overnight.

The next morning, which was Sunday, we went back down the mountain to the Quisquaia Mission Church, but because we didn't know when the service started, we were a half hour late. After church, we went to a restaurant called 'Chez Tony's', and it was terrible, but we went there because it was a fairly safe and cheap place to eat. I tried some goat dish, and it wasn't too bad.

August 4, 1986

Today, Monday, we went to the US Embassy to try to get a visa for Dieu-donnez to go to the States with Flo, to have his eyes looked at, hoping to prevent blindness like his father's. The Embassy is right in the heart of the city, and we got there at 7 am, but didn't get him in until 9:30, and that was only after Susie and I went in to ask about it, after they said they wouldn't see anyone else that day. They finally took him in after we told them his story, and showed them his passport. Flo, Dieu-donnez, and Susie were waiting inside, while Kathy, Alice, Pastor Livingston, and I, waited outside.

We waited for four hours before they finally came out again. The Embassy had told them, they needed a paper with a diagnosis from a Haitian doctor. We were encouraged by this, and Tuesday, Pastor Cebien, the pastor that Kathy and Alice work with, took him to the doctor and got the paper with the diagnosis, which we took back to the Embassy at 1:30pm. About 2 o'clock, they came back out, saying he could have a visa, but that he would still have to wait before they would give it to him. Praise the Lord!

Pastor Livingston, Dieu-donnez's dad, said his whole church was praying all week that God would make it possible for this little boy to go with Flo. I know his father was so happy, but I also know he will miss that little boy very much; he is the one who helps his father with everything, and leads him everywhere, even onto the bus, and down into the city.

On this trip, Pastor Livingston said that someone on the tap-tap had stolen his money. That's really pretty low, stealing from a blind man. He is a very sweet godly man, and his son is a sweet, quiet, shy little boy who is so excited about going to the U.S. with Flo. Nothing this good has ever happened to them before, so to suddenly have so much is really overwhelming. Flo bought Dieu-donnez some new jeans and a new shirt, and he just smiled and smiled the sweetest smile. He's such a good little boy.

We went to a big pharmacy downtown, and the area around it was unbelievable. There were wall to wall tap-taps, and people. The noise and the smells were overwhelming, and I couldn't believe what I was seeing! I don't know how Alice managed to drive there; vehicles pass each other with no more than two or three inches to spare. Flo likes to go to this pharmacy because she can buy in very large quantities and save money.

We stayed the third and fourth nights at the Overseas Mission Society compound, and it was nice, but the road we had to travel was another that defies description, but I will try.

Two lanes turned into four at times, three all the time, with two sometimes; not because there were four or three lanes ever, but that didn't bother anyone at all. It was solid like this all the way to town. We heard that on Monday night, a tap-tap had hit a man, and killed him. The people there went after the driver, but he ran and got away, so the people burned the tap-tap to a crisp. We saw it sitting by the side of the road.

Oh, yes, and weaving in and out on foot in this traffic, you have women with large loads on their heads, dogs and kids all darting in and out and around it. It's mind blowing when you see it, you don't know what keeps them all from being killed.

When we finally headed home, we stopped and bought four watermelons, and three avocados. Alice drove (thank the Lord) as Flo was very tired. All of this must be very tiring for her. I know it was tiring for me, and I'm twenty years younger than she is.

In one village, we ran into a real traffic snarl. While we were sitting and waiting for things to move, a tap-tap right next to us, but going the other way, was also stopped. Susie looked over at it, and the driver made a face at her, and said, "Boo!" Then he laughed! Susie laughed, and when I looked over, he did the same thing to me. It was pretty funny! There were people weaving in and out of the snarl with baskets full of all kinds of food to sell.

We got home about 7pm, and I was very thankful to the Lord for bringing us through all of that safely! I'm sure we had looked death in the face more than once.

August 6, 1986

Susie and I arrived at the clinic about 7:30 this morning to find moms and babies lined up and waiting. As we were watching them do triage and give out the numbers, Susie said, "Look at that tiny baby!" I looked, and saw a man holding a very small baby. I asked Ronnie to tell him to bring the baby to me, and when he did, I could see that it was a preemie – looking almost moribund. I asked the dad to let me take the baby into the clinic where I could examine him. The baby's clothing consisted of a very wet three corner diaper, made from an old sheet, a little cotton undershirt, pinned at the back to fit tightly, and a dress about three sizes too big over that. On his head was a dirty white cap, and on his feet, dirty red and white booties, about five sizes too large.

I listened to his chest, and his breath sounds were clear, but I could count every rib he had. I didn't hear a patent ductus, and except for being so skinny and wasted, he didn't look too bad. His fontanel was sunken, and the sutures of the skull were over riding, indicating dehydration, and his eyes were infected and draining slightly. I did a dextro-stick, and was not surprised to see how hypoglycemic he was. I found a feeding tube and gave him some Lytren which he tolerated. About a half hour later I gave him 15cc, or a half ounce, of some half-strength formula, praying that the Lord would just touch that tiny body. He kept it down, and everyone crowded around to see him as he slept. His eighteen year old mother had given birth six to eight weeks early, and he was now two weeks old. I wondered how he had survived for those two weeks and decided it was only by the grace of God. His mother is very sick, with a high fever and pain, and couldn't nurse him any more, which is nearly always a death sentence for the baby. The dad looked much older, though he may be the grand-father.

After we had treated the mother, we told the dad to take her home, and put her to bed, and we would take care of the baby in the clinic until we were through, or about 2pm. When the dad came back, we asked him if we could take the baby home for a few days to see if we could get him to eat. The dad said, "Thanks be to God, yes, you can." So – I went to the clinic a nurse, and came home, a 'mom'. I could hardly wait to give him a bath, and put some clean clothes on him. His name is Jean Noile, so we call him Ti-Jean, or Little John.

Susie and Anne went to Diana's and she gave them some little shirts, a box of Pampers, a stack of brand new cloth diapers, and about six pair of little sox. She also gave him a wrapping blanket, a sheet, and two little stuffed toys. Then the two girls went down town and bought a banana bark baby basket with handles. I borrowed the pillow from Flo's rocking chair for a mattress, and now, he has a sweet, clean little bed. I was just going to put him in one of my dresser drawers, but this is so much nicer. We gave him a bath, put clean clothes on him, and he looks so cute in his little bed. We were having so much fun – like playing dolls with a real live doll.

He has a great pair of lungs, but his stomach is another story. He is so malnourished that he may not be able to tolerate formula, and we don't have the right food for a starving baby. He keeps bringing the formula up, and though I think he must be keeping some of it down, it's probably not enough. He really needs to be on an intravenous hyperalimentation, and then he might make it - but we don't have any.

I gave up on trying to save him some calories by using a feeding tube, because he fights it so much, and gets all upset, which probably uses more calories. He does have a strong suck, so I guess we'll just nipple him. I'll have to set an alarm to get me up in the night to feed him. I hope we can both make it. *"Oh, Lord, may Your will be done for this tiny lamb."*

August 7, 1986

Well, I was up at 1:30am, and again at 5am. I gave him Lytren at 5, and he kept it down, so at 8, I went back to the half strength formula.

About 10am, we all left for a clinic in a village called Limonade. We were late in leaving as the house was like Grand Central Station this morning. Someone had cut our water pipe with a machete, so our cistern was dry, then a Haitian pastor stopped by to tell us of his father's symptoms, and get some medicine for him.

Then a man the missionaries call, 'Papa Noel' came by to see what Flo might need. He goes around to all the missionaries, finds out what they need, goes back to the States, and begs for what they need. He calls himself, 'the begger', but he usually comes back with the things they've asked for, and today, he had some things for Flo. He brought her a new gas cook stove for the kitchen. Now Ma'Louis will have four burners instead of two!

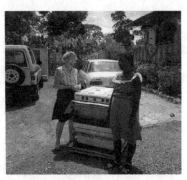

Flo and Ma'Louie with Flo's new stove.

Next, a man came by selling baskets. It was a three ring circus, but we finally got away and headed for Limonade, but the clinic had not been announced in church on Sunday, so no one knew about it, so no one was there. We all got back in the Rocky, and went home, only to find the washing machine had broken, and Ma'Louie had to finish the wash she had started in the machine, by hand. Oh, yes, one more thing. The candle I kept for a light in the bedroom last night, melted, ran all over the dresser, down the front of the drawers, and into the open drawer at the bottom, and all over about four pair of the baby's sox. What a mess!

Ti-John is still spitting. I found a small bottle of elixir of Donnatal, and I'm hoping that might settle his stomach before I feed him. So far, after two feedings with it, no difference. He's really a good little fellow, and the star of the house. Everyone who comes over wants to see 'our baby'. I just realized that he was born the day after I arrived in Haiti. *"What is Your will, Lord?"*

August 8, 1986

Today, we went with Pastor Dorléon to his village for a clinic. Susie, Anne, Ronnie, and I. Pastor Dorléon drove the Rocky through Plaine du Nord, onto a two lane dirt road, then to a one lane dirt road, to a cowpath, crossing several small rivers en route. By this time, the road had disappeared, and we couldn't drive any further.

We parked the Rocky in a banana grove, got out, and loaded all the boxes on the heads of people who were waiting there for us.

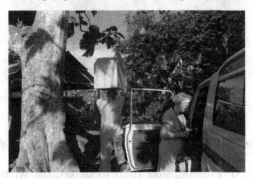

As far as we could go in the Rocky

Then, we set out on a footpath through the trees, and walked for a half an hour. It was a primitive and beautiful area – yet, there are always people. The houses we passed were all thatched roof huts with dirt floors. There was a lot of cooking going on out of doors, and our passing through was a big event!

This is truly an event oriented culture. Anything out of the ordinary in their day, is a reason to stop whatever they might have been doing, and go see what is happening. They have no entertainment, such as a radio or TV; they don't even have a clock, so whatever time you get somewhere is the right time, especially if something different happens on the way that must be investigated.

We passed a pretty waterfall where two naked little boys were playing, and unknowingly getting clean in the process; there were also fruit trees along the way, as well.

Pastor Dorléon said the name of his village was Belle Aire, and that he, and all his family live there. When we arrived in the village, there were already many people waiting for us. Pastor Dorléon had woven coconut fronds together to make walls for the clinic, and inside these walls, was a small table, a bench, and one chair. Those who were waiting sat in the open air church on what passed for pews, a board between two stumps. All of the clinics are planned with a Haitian pastor, and are held at their church. While the people wait, they sing some songs, and then the pastor preaches while we see the sick. They are sort of what you might call a captive audience, but this is the main reason for having the clinics, evangelization.

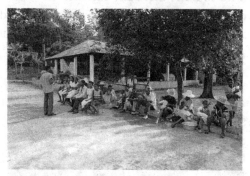

Pastor Dorleon and the beginning of our crowd.

I again played 'Doctor', and tried to determine what the problems were. I wrote notes for two to go to Limbé hospital for chest x-rays, as I suspected TB. When we send someone to the doctor anywhere, we have to give them enough money for the tap-tap so they can get there, and home again.

There were lots of folks with the usual 'traveling gas' and arthritic pain in old bones that have worked so hard at the difficult task here, of just staying alive. Such precious, sweet people. One old fellow was wearing shoes made from inner tubes, and old tire tread for soles. Ingenious! Nothing is wasted here. If it can't be eaten, they will make something useful out of it.

In the back country, most of the children have seen very few 'blancs', and some were afraid of us, crying and clinging to mom when I put my stethoscope on their chest to listen. Several women were dressed in black, mourning some relative who had died, and our last patient of the day was a lady who had two pieces of cloth pinned to the front of her dress; one was red, and the other was blue. When Susie saw it, she said to Pastor

Dorléon, "That's her problem, right there!" They had been pinned on her by a voodoo witch doctor to ward off evil spirits. She was embarrassed, and took them off, laughing as though they meant nothing, but she had gone to the witch-doctor before she came to see us. I guess his medicine wasn't working.

We saw about fifty patients, and ran out of some medicines. When we got home, Flo was very glad to see us, as she had been baby-sitting our baby, Ti-John, and was very tired.

She'd also had a meeting with the Haitian clinic workers to tell them that the clinic at Providence Orphanage would be closing when she left for her vacation, and would not re-open. She felt very bad telling them that, as for most of them it means no more jobs, so no more money to buy food.

Ti-John is still spitting, and now he is also having many loose, watery stools. I'm afraid we are not gaining any ground with his problem, and I don't know what more we can do for him. Poor little fellow. Soy formula might be what he needs, and I have none.

August 9, 1986

I decided to start an IV on Ti-John, but I only have one bag of solution, and not enough Ampicillin for a ten day course. He only keeps down about one out of three feedings, and stools constantly, so, I've decided to take him to Limbé hospital, and ask one of their doctors to care for him.

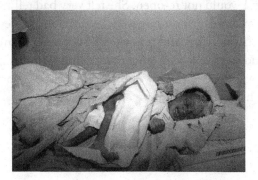

Our poor little Ti-John.

I went out to the airport to get our mail, and hopefully to see Dr. Hodges from Limbé, but he wasn't there. We nearly started a riot with Ti-John in his basket. The Haitian people have so few things of interest in their lives, that they are drawn to anything new or different, and Ti-John was certainly that! Most had never seen a baby that small, and certainly not a black baby being carried around in a basket by a 'blanc'. Finally, when I walked through the crowd in the airport, I put a cloth diaper over his face, so no one could see him, and managed to get through.

I took him out to Limbé Hospital, and had to leave him there for IV therapy. I put him into the hands of a very nice, young American doctor named Steve James, who came over from his house to see him, as no one works there on Saturday afternoon. On Monday, if the mom is better, and comes to the clinic, I'll take her to Limbé, and hopefully, she can stay with her baby and breast feed him again. I hated to leave him; the ward was so dark, with dirty looking gray blankets on little wooden cribs, sitting on an unpainted cement floor. Some of the older babies were sitting on the floor with plates of rice and beans that they were eating with both hands. Rice and beans were everywhere.

I hope he doesn't catch something else there. It's a sad place, but they do the best they can, with what they have; at least they have doctors, and a lab, so maybe they can find out exactly what Ti-John's problem is. We will be praying for this tiny person, that the will of the Lord will be done, even in this little life.

On our way home, we stopped at a house in Limbé to see Susie's little friend Marc, and take him a pair of shoes she had bought for him. It had rained a bit, and we trooped down a muddy path to Marc's house. Again, mud walls, dirt floor, thatched roof, with others like it all around. We caused quite a stir, and they all wanted to come inside the house to see what we were doing there. There was nothing but a chair in one room, and a hanging curtain separated the area, behind which, there was a bed, and that was all the furniture there was; a naked baby was sleeping on a towel on the dirt floor. Susie talked to the mom with Ronnie translating for her, and when we left, everyone followed us to the Rocky.

I have to say, a night of unbroken sleep will be a treat. I thank the Lord for Ti-John, and just put him in the hands of the One who created him, and who loves him far more than we do, though we love him a lot! I paid twenty dollars for a big box of Pampers for him. Most babies here don't wear any diapers at all.

Our washer is still not working, so four of Kathy and Alice's orphan girls came to do our washing by hand today. When they were finished, they forgot to turn off the water, so tonight our cistern is empty – no shower. Oh, well.

August 11, 1986

Today is another clinic day. Only one more day at Providence, and then it closes for good. Ti-John's mom and dad were there bright and early, and through Ronnie, I explained what I had done. I wrote them a note, gave them tap-tap money, and sent them on to Limbé Hospital.

We saw over seventy patients this morning, and again the electricity was off, so we had no fans, and no lights in the pharmacy. Today is also Susie's last day, she goes home tomorrow. I will miss her very much.

One little boy today had on a necklace of beads, shells, and some kind of teeth; probably some voodoo charm. We see a lot of babies with red thread woven into a bracelet around their wrists, and today, another child had a row of glass beads pinned inside her dress; all voodoo charms.

August 12, 1986

We got Susie off on MAF about 11.30, and then went to see how Ti-John was doing in Limbé. When I saw him, I wished I hadn't left him there. I know they try, but he was in an old, box type incubator, with a lid that lifted, and when I opened it, a bug ran under the hinge. The baby had on a gray, dirty diaper, and was lying on what looked like a bundle of old rags. He did have an IV in his arm, but he looked worse than he did when I brought him in. I was really depressed after seeing him. I really wonder just what is wrong with him, it might be something untreatable, or it just might be that he went too long without treatment, before he was brought to the clinic. This happens much too often.

August 13, 1986

It was our last clinic day at Providence Orphanage, and we saw some really sick kids. One baby had a big hole in his outer thigh; an infection from a shot given at the hospital in Cap-Haitien; unfortunately, this is quite common.

A sixteen year old girl had a terrible infection in her hand, and her fore-finger looked gangrenous. Another sixteen year old girl had a gran-mal seizure in the clinic yard before we even got started. She had been out of medicine for a week.

Flo lanced an infection in a little boy's finger, and then we saw a woman with an ear ache. When I looked in her ear, I was shocked at what I saw. There was a rotting leaf curled up in her ear, put there by the witch doctor. When I told her what was in her ear, and asked if the witch doctor had put it there, she said, "Oh, no, he just passed it over my ear." Well, when I finally got it out, I showed it to her. It had caused a bad infection in her ear – no wonder she had an ear ache!

One of our Haitian workers kept giving shots in the babies buttocks. I had told all of the workers to ONLY give babies a shot in the anterior thigh, and I had already told this girl three times, so I told Ronnie to tell her that I was watching, and if she did it again, she would be fired, so she finally got the message, I hope.

We had been seeing patients until about 2:30, when Anne came in and said that Pastor Pierre from Providence Orphanage was outside with four new padlocks in his hands. We were afraid that he would lock up the clinic, and we wouldn't be able to get all of our medicines out, so we decided to move them all right then.

In the course of going back and forth from the clinic to our house with medicines, another pastor stopped us and wanted to talk about having a clinic at his church, so we had to take the time to talk to him. Then, there was a fellow in and out of our house trying to fix our washer. The wind blew the orphanage gate into the side of the Rocky, and put a dent in it and knocked off some paint.

When I opened one of the stored boxes, I jumped a mile – there was a tarantula in it! I found something longer than my fingers, and opened it again, and much to my relief, - the spider was dead!

This has been a very exhausting day and we are all so tired. We finally got to bed at mid-night. After we moved all of our things from Providence, we had to pack for a clinic tomorrow at Limonade. Our living room looks like a disaster area. I wonder how many spiders we brought home?

August 14, 1986

We got up early, and drove to Limonade for a clinic at the Baptist church there. Flo, Anne, Ronnie, and I, went with only a couple of boxes of medicines in the Rocky. After a good jouncing over the road, we arrived to find over 100 people there waiting for us.

It took some time to get things organized, but we finally got it moving. We were doing well – we thought – until Flo went out to give out some more numbers, and was mobbed. She wasn't able to get any cooperation from the people, so she just decided to leave, and threw all the numbers into the air, and said she was leaving!

We couldn't do anything to dissuade her from doing that. The people became very angry, and it turned into a very bad situation. I kept wondering, *"How are we going to get out of this mess?"* I was a bit afraid that people, who were so disappointed – who had been waiting all morning, and now were refused – might become slightly ugly. But, instead, when they saw us packing up to go, they just wearily left. I felt so bad for them, especially the poor, little old ones. They would have been happy just to get some aspirin and some antacid, and now, they were denied even this. Poor, poor people.

We talked to the pastor, and finally came to an agreement. Next Thursday, Anne, Ronnie, and I will go back, and hopefully, it will work out better. We all came home feeling very rung out. These last two days have been real killers!

When we got home, Ma'Louie said that there was a sick man in the bedroom. It was one of the young men in the latest team from a church in the States, come down to help in any way they can. He was really sick with a high fever, bad stomach cramps, vomiting, and diarrhea. He was moaning, holding his belly, and hyperventilating. Nothing would stay down, so when Flo finally found the emergency box in the mess in the living room, she gave him a shot which quieted his stomach, so we could finally get some medicine down him.

He was on MY bed, so I slept on a roll-away bed in Flo's room. That's the way the day ended, and it started with our finding that all of the money from yesterday's clinic at Providence Orphanage had been stolen. We forgot to bring it home, and someone broke in and took it.

August 15, 1986

After a cup of coffee and a cinnamon roll, (Ma'Louie makes them, plus two loaves of fresh bread every week; we're really suffering here, poor missionaries!) I decided to tackle the front room, and see if I can bring some order out of chaos. It is a very large front room, and it's nearly filled with boxes, three deep! No order IN the boxes either. Each box has a variety of everything imaginable in it.

I wondered, yesterday, how many spiders we had brought home – well, today, I found out! When one tried to get away, I hit it with a fly swatter, and I couldn't believe my eyes! It looked like it exploded! A thousand baby spiders ran in every direction! I was swatting everywhere, trying to kill them all. I opened every box with much caution, after that, and was rewarded by finding several more good sized fellows.

Dr. Harry Davis and his wife Ann came by, and he said that they might be able to go to Limonade with Anne and I on Thursday. Praise the Lord! That will be wonderful!

It's always good to have a man along for crowd control, especially one who is also a REAL doctor!

Our house patient was somewhat better today. He finally got up, took a shower, and ate some soup, so I guess I'll have my bed back tonight.

I worked for ten hours on the boxes, and it's still a big mess, but I'm making headway. I cleaned my room, and my bed, took a cold shower, and I'm very tired tonight.

I had a good talk with a Haitian Christian named Wilber, today. He's a sweet young man who really loves the Lord. I had given him John's tape on "The sufficiency of Scripture", and he liked it, so I gave him another to listen to. Alice and Kathy are listening to "The Lord's Prayer" album, and they love the teaching. They've made two trips to Port-au-Prince in two days, still working on Dieu-donnez's visa, and have been listening while they travel. They keep coming back, and saying, "Can we have the next one?" It makes me happy to be able to put this good teaching into the hands of these very special people, and share the joy I feel when I listen to God's word expounded in a way that truly glorifies the Lord,

116

and enlightens the listener. I would love to start a tape ministry here for 'hungry Christians.'

It rained tonight, and was SO loud on our corrugated tin roof, that I couldn't go to sleep. I guess it was a good thing I was not asleep, because about mid-night someone came and asked me to come and give a shot to one of the team's boys who was sick, so I got up, got dressed, and went and gave him a shot. I hope he will be well enough to go home in the morning with the rest of his team.

August 16, 1986

Only two more days before Flo leaves for her two month vacation in the States. She is still waiting for the visa for Dieu-donnez to go with her. Flo, Kathy, and Alice will go to Port-au-Prince on Monday, and if they don't get it then, he won't be able to go. The Lord knows, and will give what is best.

Went to the airport today for the mail, and I received a letter from Dr. Benson that was a deciding factor for my not going with Medical Ambassadors.

I worked all day again, sorting things in boxes, with constant interruptions. Wilber, Ronnie, a pastor wanting a clinic, a woman selling onions, Roseanna (a cute little old man, who comes by periodically for a bag of food), one of the team fellows, and our patient, Robert, was back to take a shower before leaving for the States and home.

A little later, Kathy and Alice came by, but I love to have them come, they are such super people, who love the Lord, and are so much fun to have around. They tell the best stories about their time here in Haiti; Alice is the comedian and Kathy is her straight man, what a team!

August 17, 1986

I stayed home from church this morning, and listened to one of John's tapes, while I continued to work sorting boxes. I'm actually getting some stacked up now, ready for Dr. Harry; some for the hospital, and some for us. Not quite so many interruptions today, but the temperature was ninety-six degrees, with a humidity of eighty percent! Really sticky!

Flo is busy packing for her trip. Anne went to church, came home, and went to sleep for three hours. We woke her up with our screaming and swatting the floor, trying to kill a two inch long cockroach that I had sprayed with bug spray, and he was frantically trying to escape.

I had a nice shower and then went to English church. While I was there I talked to Faith who was taking care of Ti-John at Limbé hospital when we went to see him on Tuesday. When I asked her how he was, she told me – he had died a few days ago. I wasn't too surprised. I didn't think that he was going to make it when I last saw him. Poor baby; how much suffering he is spared now that he is in the best place there is – Heaven, held in the tender arms of Jesus, never to know sickness or hunger again.

August 18, 1986

Another day spent sorting boxes. Today, I have to admit I am beginning to get a little tired of doing this. We took several boxes to Dr. Harry's house, and a few to Jerry for her clinic, so at last, the floor is within sight again.

Flo, Kathy, and Alice went to Port-au- Prince again today, still trying to get Dieu-donnez's visa so he can go with Flo. They didn't get home until 9:30pm tonight, but, praise the Lord, they finally got it! Dieu-donnez will be able to have his eyes taken care of now. Flo said how often she has seen the Lord wait until the eleventh hour to answer a request. It was a lesson of waiting in faith for all of us. God is SO good, and with Him, nothing is impossible!

August 19, 1986

I took Flo to the airport this morning, and we waited and waited, and finally Kathy and Alice came, bringing Dieu-donnez and his mother. His older brother, Caleb, had to ride the tap-tap, as there wasn't enough room in the car for him. They have been telling Dieu-donnez to 'stick to Miss Flo' so he wouldn't get lost, and as soon as he got to the airport, he started 'sticking'. He never left her side for a minute. He was so excited, and very scared. This is the most exciting thing that has ever happened to him in his short life.

When we had gotten Flo and Dieu-donnez aboard the plane, and they had taken off, we drove to a place called Labadee. The road there could hardly be called a road, and it cost each of us $3.00 just to get in, but it was worth it. It has a beautiful white sand beach, and a beautiful clear water cove. Since it was Alice's birthday, we felt she deserved a treat, and we all enjoyed Alice's birthday.

When we came back to the house, we didn't stay long, but went to another missionary's beautiful house on the mountain, and ate hot dogs, and homemade ice-cream. Poor missionaries, my foot!

August 20, 1986

I spent the day moving into, and really cleaning Flo's room. Now Anne and I each have our own bathrooms. The two girls from the orphanage came and washed all the sheets and towels in a big pan outside. It took them about five hours, and they earned $2.00 each, which is very good money for Haiti. (I also gave them a jar of peppermints.) Ma'Louie hung the wet clothes up on our clothesline in the back of the house, and later took them all down, folded them, and put them all away. She mopped the bedroom floor, (ceramic tile) and cleaned the bathroom. When I asked her to 'shake' the rugs, she thought I said, 'wash' them, so poor Ma'Louie washed those big rugs in a BUCKET, and then hung them on the line! I felt really bad about that!

After dinner, Anne and I spent the evening getting our medicines ready for the clinic in Limonade tomorrow. Dr. Harry Davis and his wife will go with us to help us. Praise the Lord! It's got to be better than the last one!

August 21, 1986

The clinic in Limonade was wonderful, very calm, quiet, and orderly! Sometimes it really helps to have the presence of a man there. Dr. Harry and I both consulted, with Ronnie translating for me, and Anne worked the pharmacy. Of course, Dr. Harry and his wife both speak very good Créole.

I had only a few patients, that I either couldn't think what to do for them or they were so sick, I sent them to Harry. The rest of the patients that I saw, I managed to diagnose, and treat myself. For two of them, I even managed to do it all in Créole. It's easier to ask the questions than it is to understand the answers, but it was a good feeling of progress for me.

When we were finished, Dr. Harry and his wife wanted to talk to me. They said that they couldn't do the clinic again, because of the way the money was handled, and because he would like to start a clinic there, and if he continued with this money problem, of giving all but ten percent to the pastor whose church we used, it would ruin whatever ministry he might have there. He feels that by doing it that way, we are paying them to let us come and help them. His feeling is that this is not good for them, and he may be right, I don't know. The politics here are sure involved! Especially for such a simple place. So – I will have to tell the pastor, when he comes for his money, that we can't have another clinic until Flo comes back, as Anne and I can't do it alone. We saw about 85 people between 10am, and 1pm.

Tonight Kathy, Alice, and a teen-ager they have visiting them, came and had dinner with us. They had to leave just before 7pm, as Kathy was needed to play the organ for the music at the Pastor's Conference that Pastor Cebien was having at his church in Morne Rouge.

August 22, 1986

I thought about my son Jim today, while we were in our clinic. (He's 34 today.)

It was a good clinic today. We saw about thirty people, with only a few really sick folks. One eighteen month old little girl, I sent to Limbé. Her face, hands, lower legs and feet were extremely edematous. I couldn't give her any medicine, as I really didn't know what was wrong with her, and I was afraid it might be a kidney problem, or kwashiorkor, a severe protein deficiency, for which I had nothing to help her. We didn't even have any powdered milk to give her.

When we got home from the clinic with Pastor Dorléon, Kathy and Alice came by to get some water from us. Those poor girls really have a hard time with just the necessities, never mind the non-essentials!

August 24, 1986

We went to Pastor Cebien's big church at Morne Rouge today, and the girls told me that he had gone to Port-au-Prince, and had not gotten back last night as planned. We found out that he was still trying to get back, and that he'd had six flat tires on the way. Poor man!

We stayed after church to visit with Kathy and Alice – what special people they are! Anne told us her story of two years as an anorexic. She said that she didn't really remember any of it, but told us what she'd been told. What an insidious disease!

We went to the evening service which was the end of the Pastors Conference. He's had over twenty pastors there for a week. He's housed and fed them all for that week. How, I don't know. A choir of about twenty ladies, and ten men, sang acappella, and I recorded some of it. It was very nice. Then, they had a drama skit with a funny story, and a moral at the end. Alice translated it all for me as it progressed, and it was funny. The congregation enjoyed it a lot! They laughed and laughed!

After the skit, Pastor Cebien preached from 10:30 until 11:30pm, and two people came forward after the service to receive Christ into their lives. Praise the Lord! Four hours of sitting on a bench about eight inches wide, with my feet dangling above the floor was very painful - but worth it all! There was a bus there to take people home, but it didn't have any headlights, so Alice had to drive ahead of the bus with her headlights, and flashers on. Anne drove the Rocky behind it. Our Rocky was on empty when we got home, but we made it.

August 25, 1986

Anne went to the beach today, after going to Kathy and Alice's to pick up four girls from the orphanage, who came here to do all of the laundry, for all of us. Kathy and Alice have to go to Port today, to take the teen-ager, who's been visiting them, to the airport to go home.

After Anne went to the beach, I started in on the mess in the living room again. Then, the electricity went off, and, the pump did too, so – no water for laundry! I went out, and took the tin lid off of the cistern, and it was full to the top. I got a bucket and the girls dipped water to do the wash, instead of turning a faucet.

Then, Ma'Louie came, but with no electricity, or water, there wasn't much she could do, so she swept the floor, and then went home again.

My first visitor was Ronnie, and we sat and talked for a while, and then the electricity came back on. Next, Pastor D'Orléon came to get his box of medicines for his clinic that I had fixed for him, and by now, it was looking like rain. Anne hadn't come back, so I sent the four girls home on the tap-tap, and kept the clothes they'd washed here.

Anne finally got home about 5pm, and loaded up Pastor D'Orléon and Ronnie, and took them home.

After they had gone, it started to thunder, and the poor dog next door was trying to get through our grill work door, he was so frightened! He belongs to our friend, Sandy, a fellow from Nova Scotia, who is working with some Haitians making wooden toys. His dog's name is Chien, or Dog. Very original! Anyway, I brought the poor dog into the house, and shoved him under the couch until Sandy got home, and came over and got him. What a day! But a very nice rain!

I found out several weeks later, that while the washed clothes were sitting outside in the basket, someone stole some of Kathy and Alice's underwear!

August 26, 1986

It was a very uneventful day until 3pm, when Pastor Cebien had made an appointment to talk to me about medicines, or so I thought. He uses herbal medicines that his grandmother taught him to make, and I thought maybe he wanted to know how I felt about them, but that wasn't what he wanted to talk about; instead, he asked me to come back and work with him in his organization, in his clinic, here in Morne Rouge.

He is a truly remarkable man, gifted by God in many ways, yet he is such a giving and humble man. I was surprised that he asked me this, and now I must prayerfully consider, is this where the Lord would have me? I have felt all along that Medical Ambassadors was just the means to bring me to this place, and then I would be told what the next step would be.

I explained to him that I must go back to California in October to report back to the elders at Grace Church. He told me that he would be passing through California in October, so in the Lord's perfect timing, we can be at Grace Church at the same time. I also told him that Grace would be having their Shepherd's Conference at that time as well, and maybe he would like to go to that. He said he would like that, and would even take the extra time away, if he could work it in. God is so good! I would love working with these three wonderful people.

"Oh, Father, You know me better than I know myself, help me to check my motives, and show me my heart. You are putting me to the test now. I said I wanted to go to the mission field; I cried and begged You to send me. Yet, while I was here, in Haiti for this time, I felt safe, knowing I would be going home after three months. Now, I must ask myself, can I really do this? Is this really the place You want me? And I must answer, "Oh, Lord, You gave all for me, can I do less for You? I only want to be what You want me to be, and only to be where You would have me be!"

August 27, 1986

I had been in bed for an hour or so, when, about 12:45, I heard a motorbike drive up the driveway and stop. Then, I thought I heard someone call, "Anne." I didn't hear Anne getting up or answering, and then at my window, I heard, "Pat". I answered, "Yes," and the voice said, "It's Ronnie, I need some help."

I got up, put on my robe, and as I passed Anne's door, I said, "Anne, it's Ronnie." She got up too, and we went to let him in. He had another fellow with him, and proceeded to tell us what had happened. His finger was bleeding, and he said he had been playing the Haitian domino game, but when he decided to quit, the fellow he was playing with didn't want him to quit, and picked up a rock to hit him with. Ronnie tried to stop him by putting his hand on the guy's forehead. The guy pulled Ronnie's hand down off of his head, and as it passed by the guy's mouth, he got Ronnie's little finger in his mouth, and bit it, going nearly to the bone. When he got it out of the guy's mouth, the guy took off.

Ronnie said he couldn't find a doctor anywhere, so he went into a pharmacy where a man poured some Haitian rum on it, and then put some tetracycline antibiotic into it, but Ronnie was afraid of infection, so he came to us.

Neither Anne nor I felt that we could stitch it, so we soaked it in betadine, and took him to Pastor Cebien. We had to untie the gate, wake up Kathy and Alice, who went and got Pastor Cebien. He came, looked at it, and went and got some dark colored liquid – something he had made, and told Ronnie to put his finger in it. Pastor crouched down on the floor, and made sympathy faces as Ronnie nearly flew up off the couch as the stuff started to burn his finger. Pastor Cebien then dried Ronnie's finger, during which Ronnie nearly wept, and then he put some antibiotic ointment on it, and wrapped it up.

He told Ronnie to leave it alone for five days, and then he said it would be well. Now, we'll see how well his medicine works.

Ronnie crashed on our spare bed, and stayed what was left of the night. His friend left.

August 29, 1986

God has brought a Maytag washer repairman here, so we finally got the washer fixed. It still needs a new belt, but he showed us how to make it work. Praise the Lord!

We made the trip to San Raphael again, only the rocky part of the road seemed even longer than it was the last time we went. We had expected Kathy, Alice, and Pastor Cebien to be at our house at 7am. By 8:30, they still weren't here, and Ronnie had gotten tired of waiting for us to pick him up, so he walked over.

They finally arrived, and just as we had gotten everything loaded into the Rocky, the little boy from the front house came running to say we had a phone call on their phone. Anne ran down the drive to get it, and we drove on down to wait for her. She came out all smiles, and said it was Flo. She had called to say that the doctors there had found nothing wrong with Dieu-donnez's eyes! They felt his problem was a psychological one; a little boy afraid, that what had happened to his father's eyes would happen to his, too.

Again, God's perfect timing! Had we gone when we planned, we would have missed the call. As it was, now we were able to tell his parent's the good news. And Flo didn't even know that we were going to San Raphael today – but God did!

Sunday, August 31, 1986

I can't believe another month is gone. I don't feel like I am accomplishing much here, but I know the Lord is, and that's what's important. Went to church at Morne Rouge again, and it was very difficult sitting on that narrow bench. No matter which way I turn, I can't get comfortable, plus, I can't understand much of the sermon, so I'm like the little kids, with my eyes wandering everywhere.

Here are some of the things I observed; a tiny girl with sticks for arms, but bright ribbons in her hair; another little girl sitting on the narrow bench in front of me. Her feet are swinging to and fro, but her fancy white shoes are sitting on the floor; an old woman, with great dignity in her face, yet touched by sorrow and pain, walks slowly down the aisle to put her tithe in the basket. She is dressed for today in an elegant black dress, indicating she is a widow; the church is decorated with long strands of toilet paper tied together at intervals to form a design. Pink, green, peach, and white squares of tissue paper cut in fancy designs, and bright pom-poms, all colors twirling on long strings under the fans, which whirr quietly, creating a most welcome soft breeze. There are a great variety of lizards climbing the walls, and a rooster walks regally down the aisle, though no one notices him, but me, the stranger here.

I came home and took a nap, as last night was a lost cause as far as sleep went. Something woke me every hour, it seemed.

Once, it was Nikki, Flo's cat. She had been sitting on the kitchen counter, below the window, trying to catch the bugs, which were outside, and flying around the outdoor light. Her claw hooked in the screen, and pulled it down, and everything came down on the floor with a terrible crash! Scared me to death! I got out of bed, walked into the kitchen, and there she sat, on the screen, looking at me as if to say, "So-o-o-!"

The dogs were barking a lot, and I got up several times to see what they were barking at, but saw nothing. Nikki wanted out, then wanted back in, while a donkey, somewhere close, sounded like he was in mortal agony. It was not a very restful night!

September 2, 1986

I went to Pastor Cebien's clinic this morning to watch him working with his patients. I dearly love this man for the Spirit of the Lord I see in him, but – I have to say, his medicine blows my mind! And yet, his patients get well, pay him well, and come back to him.

One lady, who probably weighed 300 pounds, came to him all the way from New York, where she now lives. And for her – he put something in her navel with camphor in it, saying that he was going right to the intestines. He is going to help her lose weight, and get rid of her insomnia, and her indigestion. (She must be digesting something!) Watching him, I really don't know what to think. He does use some drama, as this makes his patients happy.

I believe the Lord is leading in this direction, but I must be able to work with Pastor Cebien, and to believe in what he does.

I saw Dr. Harry today. He told me on Sunday that they thought they would have to give up on a clinic themselves, but that today, it looks as though they will be able to start one if they can find a building. I'm sure the Lord will bring it all together for them, if that is His will. That's one reason why we do it through a local church. Besides having the patients who are waiting, hear the Gospel, it also takes care of the problem of where to have it.

We went to a Bible study tonight, but the leader was another 'prosperity' preacher, telling everyone, "to claim things from God." His message was, "Tell God what you want, and He must do it for you. Tell Him what kind of house you want, and then He has to get it for you, - even if the house belongs to someone else!"

What effrontery! What presumption! As though God was a genie, just there for our benefit, instead of us being created for His benefit. I'm so thankful for the good, straight, Bible teaching I've been privileged to have, to know Him for Who He is, and He is NOT our slave, but rather, we are His. He is the only great and glorious God, who alone is worthy of praise and glory! That alone is the only reason He gives us breath, to praise Him and lift Him up – not to tell Him what to do, as though we were the omniscient ones! I could hardly sit still and keep quiet. Sometimes, I wonder if I should.

September 3, 1986

Finally! Praise the Lord! I finally finished that front room! It still looks a bit cluttered since I still have boxes piled here and there, one for Harry, one for Limbé, one for Pastor Cebien, and one to go out in the shed. I just hope it all fits.

Now, my next project is – to make twenty-six skirts for Kathy and Alice's girls to wear for school. Someone gave them thirty yards of blue cotton material, so they sent it home with me, and a sewing machine the other day. Once I get this finished, if I ever do, then I can concentrate on the clinics. Oh, well, "Whatsoever thy hand finds to do, do it with all thy might, and as unto the Lord!" Eccl. 9: 10 KJV Amen!

We are planning to go to the Citadel tomorrow. Hope I can make it up the hill.

September 4, 1986

Ronnie's aunt forgot to wake him this morning, so we waited a half hour for him, and then came home. He showed up about an hour later, all apologies, and very upset. We told him it was OK, we'd try again next week to go to the Citadel. So – I put them both to work, hauling out the boxes I had ready, and delivering them to everyone.

The front room is beautiful now! I put the sewing machine against the wall, and folded all that material. I'm ready to start soon on that project. I may try to hire a Haitian lady to help me, as I'm afraid it may take all my time.

September 5, 1986

We made the trip to Belle Aire for a clinic today. I must be ageing fast, as that walk seems longer every time I make it. It was so hot this morning, that by the time we arrived, we were dripping!

We got started about 9:30, and by 10:30, we had seen only five people. By 3pm, we had seen fifty people. Actually, more than that, as sometimes we saw two or three people on one ticket.

One mother came with a year old baby with hydrocephalus. It's head was so large, she could hardly hold it, and she wanted me to fix it. I drew pictures of what was happening inside the baby's head, and had Ronnie explain the pictures to them, so they would understand why I couldn't fix it. I wrote her a note to take to the doctor at Limbe, but I didn't think he could fix it either. It needed a drain put in, to drain the fluid from the head to the abdomen where it would be absorbed by the body. It was very sad.

I also wrote a note for another lady who had a large growth on her 'Adam's apple'. It was as large as a tennis ball, and I had no idea what it might be.

One little boy came with an ear ache, and when I put the otoscope in his ear, I gasped. I couldn't believe what I saw! No, not a curled up leaf this time, but hundreds of tiny flies, crawling around in his ear! I said, "Anne, come and look, and tell me what you see."

She looked, and said, "Ugh! I don't believe it!" We managed to get all the flies to leave by gently patting the side of his head for a few minutes while they all flew out. Then I put some antibiotic ear drops in his ear, and then some cotton, so nothing else could get in. I gave his dad some antibiotics for him, some vitamins, and some Vermox for worms, and sent him on his way.

We give all the children Vermox, as they all have worms, and today, it seemed that everyone, young and old, had worms. We ran out of Vermox, and had to use another worm medicine, piperizine. I feel like we should just come and de-worm the whole village.

We got home about 3:30, and we were tired! I cooked dinner, and Anne did the cleanup. Then we sat down, under the fan and read, in our nice clean front room, that Ma'Louie had cleaned while we were gone. It was a joyous day, even though we were hot, tired, and sticky. The Lord is so good, and He blesses me far above what I can ask. I will never feel adequate to the task, but "His strength is made perfect in my weakness."

September 6, 1986

The mail plane didn't come until 2pm, as they went to Port-au-Prince first today, so I got some washing and ironing done. When we went to the airport, I had only two letters. One letter from my Kathy, and one from Dr Benson, telling me that he would be in Port on the twenty-third of this month. I don't know what I will tell him.

Sunday, September 7, 1986

We went to church this morning at Morne Rouge, and after visiting with Kathy and Alice afterward, Anne and I went to Mont Jolie Hotel for lunch. There is a nice swimming pool, so she went swimming, and I nearly had a heatstroke, waiting for her to finish. These last three days have been extremely hot!

We went to English church this evening, and I took my fan – it was SO hot! Occasionally, a tiny breeze would come through the window, but riding on it was also the smell of the bay, which is an open sewer. Hope it's a little cooler tomorrow!

September 8, 1986

I spent the day with Pastor Cebien in his clinic, watching him diagnose, prescribe and treat people. He saw children to very old people.

One lady told him she had been poisoned, as her husband's ex-girl friend was angry about her marrying him. Another poor woman had been hit in the face by a fist, and I think her jaw was broken. It was very swollen, and she could hardly talk, and was in a lot of pain.

At 12:30, I went home and had some p-nut butter and jelly, and then went back to watch him making his medicines. We went into a big room, and on a table were all kinds of plant stems and leaves. Over a charcoal fire, a huge cast iron pot, was set to boil. He showed me the various leaves, some of which I knew, and told me what they were used for. Then, he washed them, and threw them in the pot to boil. Then we went to make up a batch of liniment for arthritis, and rheumatism.

I can't believe I'm doing this, and I was saying that I knew I'd be ostracized by any medical people, but I really believe in this man, and his medicine. Kathy and Alice swear by his cough medicine, and say it really works!

He kept calling me, "My Sister," today, and it really tickles me. Only in Christ can we truly be all members of one body, and one family, no matter what color we might be. It's not the color of our skin that matters to God, but the color of our hearts, whether they are black or white. If it is black because of sin, the only way it will ever be white is by each person giving his heart to the Lord Jesus Christ for cleansing.

September 9, 1986

Cooler and windy today, there is a storm in Puerto Rico. I made one skirt, and probably could have made more, but the electricity kept going off. I took it to Kathy and Alice's, and tried it on four year old Magdala, and it fit her OK. I had trouble figuring out how Alice's sewing machine worked, but I finally got it to go.

This evening, Anne and I walked up to some old ruins of what probably was an old sugar plantation house. It is way out behind our house. We picked up some pottery shards that looked like very old patterns, and I wondered if perhaps some elegant French plantation owner might have eaten off of them in the years before the revolution here.

The walls were covered with vines, and were only partially intact, but it had been a big two story house. I wish those old walls could talk and tell me what happened there, and when. I wonder if it was during the slave rebellion. No one here today seems to know. Its history is forgotten.

September 18, 1986

I must try and bring this up to date. In Pastor Cebien's clinic on Thursday, a little girl, maybe two, or two and a half years old, was brought in, and she looked moribund. She was rigid, semi-comatose, teeth clenched, decerabrate posturing with her hands, and she was foaming at the mouth. Her mother said that she hadn't eaten for three days. Her cry was abnormal, and her only response to stimuli, was to go into spasm. I thought she must have meningitis or tetanus, but the mother blamed the grand-mother, and said that she was trying to kill the child by poisoning her. Pastor Cebien didn't believe that, and started to work on her.

The first thing he did was to put some of his potent nose drops in her nose. That sent her into another spasm. Then, he began to put the same medicine into her mouth through her clenched teeth, and I was afraid that she would aspirate it, but she didn't. Every fifteen minutes, he put more into her mouth, and massaged her throat to get it to go down.

When she had relaxed a little, he told the mom to take her out to his waiting area, and keep putting the drops in her mouth every fifteen minutes. Then he had someone fix a basin of very hot water, and he put some of the same medicine into it, and told the mom to put the child across her lap with her face over the steam coming off of the basin, so she would breathe it. I took a whiff of it, and it cleared my sinuses from my head to my toes!

I looked out once to see how she was doing. She was sitting up, looking around, and now they were bathing her with the mixture in the basin.

By noon, which was about three hours from the time she arrived, she was alert, crying normally, and was asking for food! It was most amazing!

Pastor Cebien said that at the next clinic on Monday, the mother came, and brought him a big bowel of rice and beans for saving her daughter.

Friday, the twelfth, we went to San Raphael, and had a good clinic, and a good dinner, thanks to Pastor Livingston's wife. I learned more about Pastor Cebien's medicines that day, as I wrote the prescriptions for him, and we had brought a lot of his medicines with us, so I had a chance to learn which medicine was used for what problem.

Saturday, the thirteenth was mail day, and I had a nice letter from Abby, in the Outreach Department at Grace Church, giving me the dates of the Pastor's Conference there, and Lord willing, Pastor Cebien will be able to go! God's timing is wonderful!

In the evening, Anne and I went to another missionary's house for pizza. About two hours after I ate it – I lost it!

I have been sick for four days. What misery! My temperature went up to 104.4, and at that point, I thought I'd better start taking something; so I doctored myself with some tetracycline antibiotic. Wednesday, I still felt terrible.

Kathy, Alice, and Pastor Cebien came by to see me, and I told him I was desperate, and I was ready to try some of his medicine. He went home and boiled up a fresh batch of something for me, and sent a bag of leaves, and some citron to make into a tea. I made the tea, and after several spoons of sugar, which he said was OK, it wasn't bad! Then I took a big spoonful of the still warm medicine, and it wasn't bad at all!

Now, I had been practically living in the bathroom, but after the first dose of Pastor's medicine, I slept all night, and have been fine since. He was so pleased that I would try his medicine, so today I drove over to show him how well it worked, and he was even MORE pleased. I was glad that I had gone, as he left about twenty minutes later on a tap-tap for Port-au-Prince.

Anne went with Dr. Harry and his wife for a clinic, but I didn't go, and I'm not going to Belle Aire tomorrow, as I'm sure I'd never make that half hour, up hill hike. I barely make it when I'm feeling strong, so I'll stay here and make skirts. I've only gotten seven made so far, but five of them had straps, and that took longer. I can make one an hour without straps. Only nineteen to go!

September 19, 1986

It was a very pleasant day today. I stayed home from the Belle Aire clinic, and made four skirts, listened to two of John's tapes, and lots of music.

Last night, after I turned off my light, out of the corner of my eye, I saw a tiny flash of light. At first, I thought it was outside, and then I realized it was a little fire fly, and he was in my room, doing spirals and loop the loops above the window. I called Anne to come and see, and she saw it doing it's acrobatics, too. I also found a tiny praying mantis in my bathroom, so I rescued him, and put him outside, where he could eat lots of bugs for us.

Tonight, there was a good sized fire way up on the mountain, but I have no idea what was burning. At home, a helicopter would have flown over, and put it out with one water drop, but here, they have nothing to fight fire with, it will just have to burn itself out. It's very dry right now, with little rain.

This evening, while Anne and I were cooling off on the front porch, we could hear many loud, angry voices across the street, and then a woman began screaming and screaming. It finally settled down again, and I hope no one was hurt. One young girl's boyfriend beat her up over there a few days ago, and I hope it wasn't her again.

As soon as a fight starts, everyone within earshot runs over to watch. It's like the special feature of the evening's entertainment. Anne and I even started down the drive to see what was going on, but about halfway down the dark drive, we decided that maybe that wasn't such a good idea after all, and we went back to sit on the porch. (Sandy told us later that sometimes they scream like that when they see a snake.)

September 20, 1986

Mail Day! No report given, on the local radio station, of any planes coming in today, but we drove to the airport about 11am, and Agape Flights came, and brought mail for us. I had told Agape Flights that I needed to go to Port-au-Prince next Saturday to talk to Al Warren, the dentist from Grace Church, who is working in Port-au-Prince. The elders want me to be accountable to him, while I am here, and I need to talk with him about coming back to Haiti, to work with Pastor Cebien. Maybe Pastor Cebien can go and talk to Al Warren, and then Al could tell Monnie what he thinks about him. They seem to be relying solely on Al's judgment, but they will be meeting Pastor Cebien at the Shepherd's Conference, and can make their own judgment then. I know the Lord will work it all out in the way that He knows is best.

Why am I even thinking about what might be tomorrow? To be anxious about tomorrow is a sin! *"Forgive me, Lord, and teach me to trust You more. Keep my eyes fixed on You, and You will keep my feet on the right path."* If it is His will, He will DO it, if it isn't His will, I don't want to do it anyway, so WHY am I fretting??

September 23, 1986

I have been sewing for two and a half days, and I only have one and a half skirts left to do. Then I have to make a button hole, and sew a button on each one and they will be finished!

This morning, I went to Pastor Cebien's clinic, and enjoyed it, but – it blows my mind! I did see the little girl I described on September 18, and she is fine. She seems and looks, perfectly normal.

Pastor Cebien has a big old yellow Toyota Landcruiser he calls the 'Lemozine'! (We all call it "The Lemonzine.") He drove me home in it, and it had to be pushed to get it started. We got out to the road, and it died. Men came running from everywhere, even from across the road, saying, "It's Pastor's car, let's give him a push!"

I just can't believe that he is going to go to the Shepherd's Conference at Grace. It's too good! He said he would arrive on the thirteenth of October at LAX, so I'm going to leave to go home on the seventh, to be ready to go get him when he arrives. God is SO good, He delights to do the impossible for His children. May He be glorified in all that happens!

September 24, 1986

Today, I went up the river from the bay, in a small outboard motor boat that Ronnie had arranged for Anne and me with some friends of his. What a trip! The river is literally a floating garbage can and latrine combined. The banks of the river are solid with garbage, and those who live alongside it build their latrines out over the river. The smell is nauseating! People live there, and little children play there.

Once we were passed the city area, I saw men fishing with nets; a few birds, lots of mangrove swamps, and tiny shacks scattered along the river banks. All I could think of was, *"Lord, please don't let me fall into that water!"* It was awful! We went as far as we could go, and came to a place where there were fishing nets spread all the way across the river, blocking any further passage. We turned around there, and went back down the river of floating grapefruit rinds, and dead animals. I did see a couple of fish jump out of the water, but Anne said they were just coming up for air!

I was very glad to be back on dry ground, although it's not very clean either.

September 26, 1986

Anne was getting the medicine box ready for the San Rafael clinic last night, and I was outside breaking up a cat and dog fight, when I heard Anne scream.

I hollered, "What's wrong?" But all she said was, "Come here!"

I ran into the house, and she and a tarantula were sitting facing each other, both of them ready to run if the other one moved at all.

She said, "I put my hand in that box to see how full it was, and that tarantula ran up my arm!" She had flung it away, and it was now sitting there, as ugly as they come, though it was small for a tarantula.

I said, "I'll call Sandy."

He came over and scooped it up, and put it outside. Poor Anne was a basket case for the rest of the evening! I would have been the same if it had happened to me!

We left this morning for San Raphael about 8am in Pastor Cebien's 'Lemozine'. It took us two hours to get there, and another half hour to get the clinic started, as he took the car somewhere to get it washed, and had to walk back, while we waited for him.

Our clinic lasted until almost 3pm. People just kept straggling in, until we finally ran out of medicine, and had to quit.

We had a nice meal prepared by Pastor Livingston's wife, saw Dieu-donnez again, and told them this was our last clinic in San Raphael. Anne will leave on Tuesday, and then I will leave on the next Tuesday. We got home about 5:30, tired, hot, and sticky, but happy! The 'Limonzine' has no air conditioning like the Rocky has, just open windows.

Pastor Cebien is going to try to get to Port-au-Prince tonight with his daughter and niece, who have been here in Cap-Haitien all week. We've been hearing about trouble in a town called Gonaives, with road blocks again; the buses were turned back, and couldn't get through, as this is the only road from north to south.

I'm glad I decided not to go to Port to see Dr. Benson. The last time he came was during the revolution. He really picks his times!

September 29, 1986

   September is almost gone! Anne leaves tomorrow, and then I will leave the next Tuesday, Lord willing!

   Anne went to Labadee with another girl, and I went to Pastor Cebien's clinic. It was a good clinic, but I got so sleepy, I could hardly stay awake, so when I came home, I went and took a nap, while Ma'Louie ironed skirts, and made dinner for us, and Kathy and Alice. We had a very loud thunder and lightning, rain storm tonight.

   Pastor Cebien called Al Warren in Port, but wasn't able to get him to arrange a time to talk. The Lord knows.

September 30, 1986

About a quarter to eleven this morning, we left to take Anne to the airport, and as we were just getting into town, we saw a crowd of bicycles coming toward us. A Jeep going in the opposite direction, motioned for us to turn around, as he came along side of us. We kept going for a way, and then we saw a large group of people, with placards and banners walking toward us.

We said, "Uh, Oh," and turned around, and headed back the way we had come. Fortunately, Ronnie was with us, and he leaned out and asked a guy on a bicycle, what was going on. He told Ronnie that it was a demonstration about the schools. The teachers want a raise from a hundred dollars a month to three hundred, and they are going to strike. We couldn't get to the airport by going through town, so Ronnie showed us a back road – rough, rocky dirt road – but we managed to get there that way, and in plenty of time, too.

Anne got to fly to Fort Lauderdale with Steve Saint. He is the son of Nate Saint, one of the five missionaries killed by the Auca Indians in the 1950's. I'm sure she will enjoy the trip.

I have had a difficult time today, trying to discourage two young people who want money. I've already given the man over one hundred dollars for his 'poor mama' who, he said, was in the hospital, and then died. Now, he, or the girl, I don't know which, want more money to go to school. I gave her sixty dollars the other day after I read a note she gave me, telling about the 'problems' they were having – no mama, no papa, etc.,etc.

I said, "No, no more money." They just hung around for a long time on the front porch, with long faces. They must think I'm the Bank of Haiti, now. They finally left, but the young man just rode up on his bicycle, so I am hiding from him. Thank goodness, the doors are all locked as I'm alone now. I wonder how long he is going to wait on my front porch.

I think I finally convinced the guy that I was NOT going to give him any more money, after he peered through my bedroom window, where I had retreated away from him. I got angry, and jumped up and said, "I'm going to get Sandy!"

I yelled out my window, "Sandy!"

I didn't know that Sandy wasn't home, but the guy didn't know that either, so he got on his bike and as he left, he turned his head and said, "Tomorrow?" And I yelled, "NO, not tomorrow!" and off he went, and he never came back.

October 1, 1986

Today, there were more demonstrations going on in Cap-Haitien. I even heard gun shots this evening, though they've said that they are only firing into the air to frighten the demonstrators into behaving. I heard that yesterday, they marched to the head teacher's house, threw rocks at his house, and destroyed his car. I don't know what he had done, or what they were doing today, but I am going to leave the clinic tomorrow, about 9am, and go and get my shopping done before they start again! School is supposed to open on the sixth, and I leave on the seventh. Only the Lord knows what will happen between now and then.

I went to the clinic this morning, but there were no patients. Pastor Cebien said that he was going to go and buy some wood to build a church for some poor people in the mountains near Gonaieves. He said that there was only a Seventh Day Adventist Church, and a Catholic Church, and that to get to an Evangelical Church, they had to walk for three hours, so he will build them one. He really loves his people; he is a real treasure!

How I praise the Lord for His own love that He gives to us His children, and He says, " By this shall all men know that ye are my disciples, if you have love one for the other." John 13:35 KJV

October 2, 1986

I went to Pastor's clinic this morning, and then at 9:30, since we had only one more patient, I told him I would go home, as I needed to fill my drinking water jugs, and I needed to go into town to get some groceries.

I got my water, and then drove the Rocky into Cap-Haitien. (It's about a four mile drive to the store.) There were partial road blocks in quite a few places, some of them still smoking, but I was able to get through. I got my shopping done quickly, and headed home, only to come to one road that was completely blocked by big rocks piled up all the way across. I sat there for a few minutes, not knowing what to do. I guess I was hoping that a group of men across the road from me would take pity on my white hair, and come and help me.

That didn't happen, so I decided all I could do was to drive over it. I put little Rocky in four wheel drive, sent up a quick prayer for help, and over I went. The group of men looked very surprised, but they weren't any more surprised than I was! It is a high car, and didn't scrape the rocks. I made it home OK, but I hope I won't have to go to town again before I leave for the States. I need to learn some alternate routes, as I'm sure there are some, but I just don't know where yet.

We heard lots of gun shots toward town last night, but none near the house. Ronnie came this afternoon, and we talked about John's tapes, as Ronnie has gotten very interested in listening to them. He told me that, while all the shooting and yelling was going on last night, he was in his own little world, listening to John!

I drove to Kathy and Alice's this afternoon, as I wanted to see Pastor Cebien before he went to Port-au-Prince. There has been a rumor that they are planning to burn down Gonaives tomorrow, and the road to Port goes right through Gonaives. We just pray that God, in His sovereignty, will keep Pastor and his family safe, and bring him back to Cap-Haitien safely on Monday. When I got to their house, he was still there, so I got to tell him goodbye, and God bless. God is still in control! Amen!

I also heard today that a policeman or soldier was shot in the head last night, and died in the hospital. I guess some of the shooting was NOT just into the air.

October 3, 1986

We had our last clinic today in Belle Aire with Pastor Dorléon, and we must have seen a hundred and fifty to two hundred people. Sixty four tickets were given out, but every one of them had at least two to five people on it. We ran out of nearly everything, and there were still people waiting to be seen. We worked for about five hours straight.

Kathy and Alice came for dinner, and afterward, we played Bible Trivia – I lost! Kathy won, and Alice was second. It was good fun, and relaxing for all of us.

We heard that a military plane came in to the airport, and unloaded machine guns for the military here; it looks like they expect a lot of trouble. In the last two nights, my Bible reading has ended with these two verses; Psalm 82:8, "All nations are in Your hands." and Psalm 83:18, ". . .You alone, Jehovah, are the God above all gods, in supreme charge of all the earth." LB Amen!

October 4, 1986

I heard two helicopters go over, very high up. I got the binoculars out, but I couldn't see any identification on them. I learned later that Haiti's total Air Force consists of six helicopters.

Ronnie came this morning about 9am, and we went into town. I wanted to go, because I still wanted to buy a dress for my grand-daughter, Sarah. I asked Ronnie to drive, as I thought, if we had to leave in a hurry, he knew the roads out of town, and I didn't. There were still some piles of burned tires, and other debris across some streets; and one street had metal car parts strewn nearly all the way across it, along with some big rocks. Ronnie had to put two wheels up on the sidewalk to get around it. He told me that two men were killed in town last night, and they just left their bodies in the street all day. He said he saw them, but didn't know why they were killed.

After Kathy and Alice got home from my house last night, they were told that one of Pastor Cebien's Bible School students, had threatened to 'get them' that night. Those two poor girls were awake all night - waiting for 'whatever' to happen! Some of the students have threatened Pastor's life, and said they were going to 'déshouké' (to cut down) him. All of this because he closed the school last year. His reason – their attitude!

Now, they have demanded a certificate signed by him, even though they've never finished the four years. He has refused to do this, so now they're out for revenge. It's hard to believe these are Christian young men, they must have been going into ministry as a means to make money, and not to preach the love of Christ!

I hope Pastor Cebien gets back as planned, so the girls won't have to be there alone again tonight.

I read this yesterday in II Thessalonians 3:3, "But the Lord is faithful; He will make you strong, and guard you from satanic attacks of every kind." LB

October 5, 1986

I read in Jeremiah this morning, "Oh, Lord God, You have made the heavens and the earth, by your great power; nothing is too hard for You!" Jeremiah 32:17, and 32:27, "I am the Lord, the God of all mankind; is there anything too hard for Me?" LB

I got to Kathy and Alice's about 9am, and we drove up the mountain, past Limbé, to go to church where Pastor Dorléon preaches. It is one church of many that Pastor Cebien has started, and built. It's a real cute cement block church with a corrugated tin roof. Some of the cement blocks have cut out designs, and they use them where the windows are. This allows them to be able to lock the doors, so no one can break in, but during the service, the breeze can blow through the windows. This is Haitian air conditioning.

This day, the Lord most graciously sent a lovely cool breeze that blew through the door and the window where we were sitting. We were sitting on long benches with desks, as most church buildings are also used as schools, run by the pastor. Every child who attends these schools receives a nourishing hot meal every school day, which for many is the only meal they have all day.

Grace Church has many beautiful things, but one thing they don't have is the magnificent view of mountains, breadfruit trees, and a shining river, way down below that I gazed out on, from my seat in the church.

Pastor Dorléon was all dressed up in a suit and bow tie, and he preached a good sermon. A lovely young Christian man prayed, and one just felt his love for his Lord as he prayed. A men's trio sang, then Kathy and Alice sang, and a young girl sang – all without any accompaniment. The girl was a bit quavery, but I felt that it was as beautiful to the ears of God, as our full orchestra and choir at Grace.

Pastor Cebien arrived during Pastor Dorléon's sermon. I saw him drive up in the Limonzine, then, he walked down the side of the mountain, out of sight, changed his clothes, hiked back up to the church, came in, and conducted a beautiful Communion service with real bread and grape cool-aid. I could understand enough of the Créole to hear him say, "Let every man examine himself," and I was glad.

After the service, we drove back to Morne Rouge, and had a very nice dinner. Pastor Cebien stayed for a meeting at the church, so he had his dinner later, and then we all sat and visited for awhile. At 7pm we went to another of Pastor Cebien's churches, one we pass on our way to Belle Aire. It was the first church he established, and he actually built it himself; he even made the clay bricks.

There was no electricity, only a Coleman lantern hanging over the pulpit. It was such a beautiful service, with wonderful music. Pastor Cebien plays the accordion, but he's never had any lessons, and since he is left handed, he only plays the bass buttons, but he still manages to make a lot of music with his method. I will forever have a picture etched in my mind of him sitting on a chair, in the soft lantern light on the platform, his accordion on his knees, his eyes closed, his nose resting on the accordion, as he played the accompaniment for those who were singing. It was so beautiful, and to add to it, you could hear his deep bass voice in a hum, and it sounded like a big pipe organ.

A group of girls got up and sang a song about what they were going to do in Heaven, all done with action. Kathy, Alice, and Pastor Cebien sang a beautiful song together, and then he preached a good sermon. What an indescribable service, and such precious people!

We are hearing that things are getting tenser all over the country. I just pray that this turn of events will not cause Grace Church to tell me that I can't return. It would break my heart, but – the Lord knows! I really love these people, especially the three at Morne Rouge. They have repeatedly been threatened, and for the last two nights, none of them have slept. I'm so glad that Pastor Cebien is back to take care of them, but I fear for him as well. The people are beginning to feel that they are free to do anything they want to do – right, or wrong. And if they want what you have, and they do, they feel they have a right to just take it.

October 6, 1986

My last day here in Haiti, and it was glorious! Thanks be to the giver of every good and perfect gift! I got up at 5:30am, and it was still dark, but so cool. I got to Morne Rouge about 7am. I went to the school rooms and took pictures of the kids, and Kathy and Alice doing their morning flag salutes. Then, I went back to the clinic, but Pastor Cebien was still asleep, though there were people already waiting for him. I then went back to the house, and sat in the rocker for awhile, until one of the girls came to tell me that he was beginning clinic.

We had a good clinic, and two of the old people that we didn't have medicine for in Belle Aire were there. Precious old couple, though she is so skinny and sick.

Then, Pastor Cebien came and told me that there was a lady outside who was dying. I went out with him to see, and I was overwhelmed by what I saw.

There she was, comatose, skin and bones – lying in a wheelbarrow! Her family had brought her to the clinic in a wheelbarrow! That was her ambulance!

They had padded it a bit with some straw mats, laid a sheet over them, and then lay her in it. Her feet were hanging over the end, by the handles, and they were very cold feet, in spite of the fact that the day was hot.

I thought, how terrible to struggle all your life just to survive, never having enough of even the barest necessities, and then have a wheelbarrow for your death bed!

Pastor Cebien mixed up some of his potent medicine, mixed it with some sour orange and honey, and began to spoon it into her mouth, but with no response. He told the family to keep doing it, and if there was any response in the next two hours to call him. They wheeled her home – and never came back. Poor old soul!

When the clinic was finished, Pastor took me out to the slums where he is building a school. It had rained recently, and there was about a foot of dirty water every where. We couldn't get all the way out to the building. We almost got stuck in the watery garbage! There was so much water, filthy, and salty from the sea, but the little kids were having a wonderful

156

time playing in it, kicking it all over each other, running through it, and then doing a belly flop, laughing all the time. They didn't have to worry about getting their clothes wet or dirty, because, they didn't have any on.

Pastor Cebien had slyly said, that 'someone' wanted to have a party for me tonight, and asked if Miss Kathy had told me. Well, if Miss Kathy had known about it, she might have told me, but of course, it was a surprise to her too. So, I went back in the evening, and took my camera and tape recorder. It was a wonderful 'unplanned surprise party' in that everyone but Pastor was surprised! But, what a joy! The three of them sang several songs, which I recorded, some of the orphans sang, Pastor sang, Kathy and Alice sang, and I recorded it all. Then he made such a sweet speech, and they gave me some beautiful gifts.

The Lord has just made every day here sweeter than the day before it. My cup surely overflows, and I sure do love these people, and I will miss them sorely!

October 7, 1986

When you fly, you realize just how big the earth really is; that is, in relation to man. Then you think about the heavens and the whole universe, and you realize how small the earth is, in relation to all of God's universe. Then, you think about God, how glorious, - and you say with David, "What is man, that Thou art mindful of him?" And, then, even farther down the scale, 'especially a little old lady, who has thrown most of her life away,' but has given to Him now, all that He chooses to give to her.

God has given me so much joy in Haiti. It has been as He has promised, ". . .pressed down, shaken together, and overflowing!" He has proven to be faithful in every promise He has given. He has kept me in safety many times, and I have felt His presence every moment.

I have to say, I have been my most miserable, physically that is; and the happiest I have ever been – all in the same place, and frequently, at the same time!

When I got up this morning, I finished my packing, and my suitcase weighs a ton! I also have two carry-on bags, my trolley, the Haitian purses with the dolls in them, a big plastic bag, and the carved table that Pastor Cebien gave me last night. It was easy at the Cap-Haitien airport, as there were many willing hands to help me. I'll manage somehow the rest of the way.

We drove the Rocky around the back way to the airport just in case there might be trouble in town. Everyone came to see me off, including Ronnie and Pastor Cebien. They stood around in that miserable hot airport for a long time, just waiting with me. When the DC-3 was ready to board, Pastor Cebien picked up one of my bags and carried it out to the plane for me. When I turned to take it from him, he kissed me on the cheek, and said, "God bless you, my sister."

I pray the Lord will send me back, and soon! I'd rather be there with them, sharing whatever may be happening in their lives, even if it's danger, than to be safe at home wondering, what's happening to them. I pray God will keep them safe under the shadow of His mighty wings, and that the angels will camp round about them, keeping out any evil that would try to hurt them. *Come soon, Lord Jesus, but until You do – please, send me back to Haiti!"*

Back in California

159

October 24, 1986

Our mighty God is indeed the God of the impossible! He did bring my Haitian brother to California! He is staying at our house with my mother and I. (I can only imagine what the neighbors are thinking when they see this tall, skinny black man coming and going with us.)

We started out the Wednesday of the Shepherd's Conference by attending a 6am elders meeting at Grace Church. Pastor Cebien spoke to them, and so did I. What a joy to have him here with us, and for them to really get to know him better. He enjoyed the Conference very much

Some of the young College Group men have shown much interest in him, and in possibly coming to Haiti next summer to help him with his Pastor's Conference in August, 1987. Praise the Lord! That would be a great blessing for all involved.

One of the young men gave Pastor an accordion, and the last Saturday of the Conference, he and I went looking for another one, as he had saved some money to buy one here. We ended up at a music store in San Fernando, and discovered the manager is one of the young men from Grace Church who sings in the Joyful Sounds group. When he found out who Pastor was, and what he wanted the accordion for, and that he was a pastor attending the Shepherd's Conference, he let him have three accordions for $200! Praise the Lord! Now, he has four accordions to take home to give to some of the other pastors there. He finally ended up with SIX accordions, and four suitcases, one filled with clothes that people had given to him.

After the Conference we went to a meeting with one of the Outreach Department elders, and a couple who have been in Haiti for twenty years with OMS. It was more of a fact finding session, than one of making decisions. Then we went to another meeting with Al Mount. I am to go before the Selection Committee again on November fifth.

It has been wonderful to have Pastor Cebien here for two weeks. We had time to talk about several issues, and time to spend in prayer together. My desire now, is to pour out my life for the Lord, working alongside this brother in Christ, freeing him to preach as he feels God has commissioned him to do, sharing his love for his people in service to them, and to the Lord.

October 28, 1986

What a glorious battle, because we always know who will win! Praise His wonderful Name! I have just been reading my journals over again, and once more I marvel at the grace of our living God. In June, I wrote what my heart's desire and my goals for my time in Haiti were, and I see that God has fulfilled them all.

1. He has definitely confirmed my call to Haiti in Pastor Cebien's request for me to return and work with him in his clinic.
2. He gave me a real insight, and sensitivity to the people.
3. He filled my heart with His love for them, especially the very young, and the very old.
4. He gave me three special friends, family really, two sisters, and a brother, all of whom gave me such sweet Christian love, that I couldn't help but love them in return.

My desire is to go back and work in the clinic, so Pastor Cebien will have more time to go and preach as he feels called to do. Planting churches is also his calling. I just want to come along side, and relieve him of some of the load that he is carrying. The Lord has given me a love for him, and for Kathy and Alice, and the thought of the four of us working together is pure joy!

I have told Medical Ambassadors that I will not be working with them, as that was the request of the elders at Grace, so now I have no mission organization for Grace to work through. I hope and pray that they might just send me out under the elders here at Grace Church. They would prefer some organization for me to be accountable to, and I agree that accountability is important, and I'm willing to be accountable to Al Warren, if that would suffice. The Lord has moved in their hearts before on my behalf, and I know He is able. But – I must be submissive to the church as well. While Pastor Cebien was here for those two weeks, they got to know him better, and that will help with their decision.

While he was here, I had a dream that we were in Haiti, working together, and trouble started again. I dreamed they killed him right in front of my eyes, and when I fell crying on his body, they killed me. Both

161

of us beheaded by machetes. It was a terrible dream, but I didn't tell him, because he believes in dreams coming true.

The elders have discussed safety issues, but . . . "I count not my life dear unto myself," and I am ready to give up my life for my Savior if He should ask it of me, but I can not stay at home to be safe. Besides, who says that it's safe here?!

Haiti is where the reality of pouring out your life really is. Every day I was there was one of joy and peace, that only God can give when you are obedient, and walking in His will, especially when you are tired, hot, hungry, and sticky. His love is so real, and to see Him working through your hands to those who have nothing, either materially or spiritually, is LIFE – real living – what the Christian life is all about! It's being able to put action in the word love. How many times have I heard John explain, love is not a warm fuzzy feeling, it is self sacrificing service to others. This is what the Bible means when it talks about Christian love.

November 10, 1986

We arrived home today from a visit to family in Tonopah for a few days. My mother wants to live in Tonopah if I go away, so we went to look at houses, but we didn't get to see all she wanted to, as she got sick. When we arrived home, as we were emptying the trunk of the car, a lady walked up and asked my mom if her house was for sale? She said she had cash, and was ready to buy. Wow! How's that for answered prayer as to what to do??!

I talked to Pastor Cebien on the phone while I was in Tonopah. He had called us at home, and was worried when he got no answer. He wanted to know how my meeting with the elders went, and was disappointed when I had to tell him that still nothing had been decided yet. I know the Lord will work it all out in His own time.

I went by Northridge Hospital and went to the Neo-natal Intensive Care Unit to see the girls I had worked with before I went to Haiti, and was astounded by the reception I received. Everybody threw their arms around me, and gave me lots of hugs! It was really nice! They also re-hired me. I have to go back to work as my money is running out. It will be 'call-part-time' so it won't be so hard to quit, when it's time to go back to Haiti.

My back has been hurting me a lot, and it's kind of a low valley point in time right now. I hope my back problem will not be something that will keep me here. I praise the Lord for all the tests and trials here, and just ask that I might quickly learn whatever it is He is trying to teach me.

November 12, 1986

Praise the Lord! He is so full of loving-kindness, as a Father with a tiny child. He knew I was discouraged, so today I received two letters from Haiti, and one from one of the men on the selection committee. It was so encouraging.

November 13, 1986

I received a letter from Pastor Cebien today, and he writes that he 'needs me', and asks me to 'please come back soon'. I pray that this test of our faith will soon be over, and the Lord will send me back to Haiti. Oh, that I may submit to it with joy, knowing that it is stretching me, and getting me ready for the larger trials ahead. I want to grow, but it's so hard to wait!

Here is something that Joni Earekson Tada wrote:

"Waiting is never easy, but God says it's best for us. Occasionally, He grabs us by the shoulders, and sits us down hard so we're made to wait, because He knows that afterwards we'll be all the more full of grace and strength to do our daily jobs." Also, the Word tells us that, "They that wait upon the Lord shall renew their strength; they shall mount up with wings as eagles. They shall run and not be weary; they shall walk and not faint." Isaiah 40:31 KJV *"Teach me Lord, teach me Lord, – to wait!*

November 18, 1986

Tonight, I lay on the altar of obedience, my heart's desire to serve Him in Haiti. I have been begging Him to send me back, but I've been unwilling to say, that I would be willing to stay here, or to go somewhere else, if God should close the door to Haiti. Tonight, I place my desire on the altar, take my hands off of it, and give it to God. I turn it loose, and pray that I will not have even the 'fondling touch', but to let go of it completely, and wait on Him.

I think of our lovely Savior praying in the garden to be released from His task, but able to say, "Not my will, but Thine be done." I have been clinging to MY desire, and not willing to give it to God, and take my hands off. Now, it's His. My heart will break, but I know I will have the joy as well, if I am obedient.

Here is something else that Joni Earekson Tada wrote:

"The message we must hear is simply this – obey. If we could only understand from this side of Heaven how necessary it is to obey . . . how it will result in eternal rewards, how Christ will get tremendous honor and glory from our right response during tough days down here on earth. If our testimony is to mean anything to God, and to others, obedience is the key."

How can I become wine,
if I object to the fingers God uses
to crush me?
J. Oswald Chambers

November 22, 1986

Yesterday was my first day back at work in the NICU since I came back from Haiti. It was fine until about 5pm, and then people started saying to me, "You're so brave to go to Haiti," and, "I've always wanted to go somewhere like that, but I'm afraid," and so on and on.

Let me say it here, - this place is the sacrifice, not Haiti; this is the frightening place, not Haiti!

My mom called and told me that Al Mount had called, and wanted to talk to me. I called him back, and I have an appointment to see Al on Wednesday. I'm afraid my attitude has been very bad lately, and I hate it! The waiting, and the longing to be in Haiti are becoming so powerful that I can't think of anything else. I am afraid – God, forgive me - that Al and Monnie are going to suggest that I should think about going somewhere else instead of Haiti, where there would be a mission board for me to be accountable to.

Why can't I feel as sure that God will do it this time? I guess when I went the first time, it didn't matter then where I went, but now, God has given me such a love for Haiti, and such a strong desire to serve Him there, I can't even think of any other place. Here, I'm just one of a very large workforce, but in Haiti – I am the workforce!

'Help me Lord to wait with patience, that I may run this race to its finish. There is nothing too hard for my GOD! Amen!'

November 25, 1986

I read this in Psalm 113:4-8

It's all about God; how great, and so high above everything He is.

"For He is high above the nations; His glory is far greater than the heavens. Who can be compared with God enthroned on high? Far below Him are the heavens and the earth; He stoops to look, and lifts the poor from the dirt, and the hungry from the garbage dump, and sets them among princes!" LB

He cares so much for the poor and the hungry that He stoops all the way down to the lowest of the low, and to those who are hungry. What a gracious and merciful God He is! He must really love Haiti, since there are so many poor and hungry people there. I long to be used by Him to help lift them up, feed them physically and spiritually, so they too, might have all the riches of heaven in Christ!

I go tomorrow to see Al Mount again, and how I pray that he will have something positive for me. I was listening to a tape by a young man, and in it he gave a definition of the word 'passion'. I knew how I felt about going back to Haiti, but I didn't know it could be described as passion. Here is the definition, and it truly describes how I feel

Passion = An inward burning desire to accomplish something for the glory of God; a desire that is so great, it cannot be ignored, a desire so vast, it cannot be denied, a desire so all consuming, you feel like you must seek it's fulfillment or else you will die. You feel you must give your life to it in the pursuit of its fulfillment. It is fanatical commitment, nothing less than self-sacrifice; it is being totally consumed in the pursuit of a goal for the glory of Jesus Christ. Amen!

All I want in my life is to be a vessel fit for the Master's use; one that will glorify Him. So – I guess it could be said that I have a 'passion' to serve Him in Haiti, because this definition just really describes how I feel. My heart is so heavy here, and I can't get enthusiastic about working here at all. Money and things mean nothing to me, only as a means to get back to Haiti. Being willing to be despised, to suffer shame with Him here, for this world is NOT our home.

"But always remember this; it is not for your own sakes that I will do this, but for mine….." Ezekiel 36:32 says the Lord. Then, I love this prayer of David's:

"I cling to your commands, and follow them as closely as I can. Lord, don't let me make a mess of things. If You will only help me to want Your will, then I will follow Your laws even more closely. Just tell me what to do, and I will do it, Lord. As long as I live, I will whole heartedly obey!" Psalm 119:31-34 LB

"Turn me away from wanting any other plan than Yours- for You have said, You will never disappoint those who trust in You. Jehovah is mine! And I promise to obey. With all my heart, I want Your blessings." Psalm 119:57-58.

November 29, 1986

I talked again with Al, hoping to hear something positive, but again, only status-quo. He called World Concern while I was there, and another secular organization, and they will respond on Monday. I tried again to make him aware of my deep feelings about going back. I even read to him the definition of 'passion' that I had heard. They are sympathetic, but not enthused about sending me back. Al said that if I decided to go on my own, they would pray for me, but that would be all. They would consider me as not being submissive to their guidance as elders. But, I feel that human men, even elders, can be mistaken sometimes, and I reminded them that they are responsible for guiding me, and will answer to God for their decisions, according to Scripture.

I worked Thanksgiving Day, and it was pleasant. I had an opportunity to talk with my little Japanese brother in Christ, and praise the Lord, he is becoming bolder in his faith, and is making a real visual stand for Christ. It's been a good and refreshing day with the Lord. My mother has been gone a good part of the day, and it's been so nice just to be alone with the Lord. How patient He is with us, as He tries to teach us the patience that will produce the endurance we need as good soldiers of Jesus Christ. *Help me Lord, to wait, and to learn.*

December 14, 1986

What a blessed day! How I love Grace Church, and John's teaching!

When I talked with Pastor Cebien yesterday, he told me that he had had some meetings at his church, and that thirteen people had been saved – including a witchdoctor! Praise the Lord!

My mother and I made another trip to Tonopah last Sunday, and stayed until Tuesday. We went house hunting again, and found a wonderful tri-level house up on a hill, for $119,000. When we came home, my mom told the lady who wants to buy her house, to make her an offer. Her house has been assessed at $135,000. They offered $125,000, and of course she turned them down. Then they said $130,000, and I thought she should have taken it then, but she kept thinking she could get more.

She mentioned this amount to the neighbor next door, and his response was, "Take it and run!" She seemed happier about it then, but didn't call the lady to tell her. The next day, the neighbor called, and told her that it was a very good price, and she should take it. She finally called the lady and told her she would take it. Now, tonight, she's again saying that, "it's too much trouble," and she's not going to move! I don't know what to say to her. It was her idea in the first place, and it really doesn't matter to me one way or the other, so, whatever she decides is fine. For my part, however, I feel that the Lord has been pretty clear in His directions, but I can't force her to be obedient, and I feel selfish in that all I want is to be in Haiti.

My Kathy called last night to say that her hands and feet were numb and tingling. My poor sweet baby! It's a fearful thing to fall into the hands of the Living God. Why do we force God's hand sometimes? He is so gracious and longsuffering, and we still push at Him. It's a wonder to me that He doesn't just wipe us all out, but instead, He loves and cares for us. Amen!

(Dec. 20: The diagnosis of Multiple Sclerosis is confirmed on Kathy with MRI. They can see the plaques on the brain. My poor baby!)

December 18, 1986

How wonderful God is – just moving things along at His own steady pace in spite of all our attempts to work it out in our own way. To see Him working where this house and moving are concerned, is marvelous! The house here went into escrow on Monday, and the bid of $113,000. on the house in Tonopah was mailed. Today, the Real Estate lady in Tonopah called to say they had accepted the bid. I know that soon He will make my way just as clear.

I just began to read Habakkuk chapter 2, and this is what I read: "But these things I plan won't happen right away. Slowly, steadily, surely, the time approaches when the vision will be fulfilled. If it seems slow, do not despair, for these things will surely come to pass. Just be patient! They will not be overdue a single day!!" Amen! How the Lord knows how to pick us up and encourage us!

I thank Him, praise Him, and joyfully wait for Him, knowing that He sees what we cannot – both the beginning and the end – and every thing in between! He is indeed Sovereign God. I believe the waiting will soon be over, and it will be even sweeter for having waited!

December 28, 1986

Another year is nearly gone. These last two months have been an agony of waiting in what has seemed like a very dark tunnel, away from the place I long to be, and away from the ones I long to be with.

I talked to Pastor Cebien, and was so sorry to hear that his wife has taken their children, and gone to the U.S. I'm not sure I understand exactly what's happened, but it doesn't sound good. I could hear the sadness in his voice, and I felt so sorry for him. I pray for this marriage, that God will heal it, and bring his family back to him. There are always two sides to every story, and maybe she was just too lonely. She lived in Port-au-Prince, and he was much of the time in Cap-Haitien, so he was away from his family much of the time, and there were four children to care for.

My poor mother continues to allow Satan to harass and upset her over this move. Again this morning, she didn't want to move. God is not the author of confusion, nor has He given us a spirit of fear. How we need to praise Him continually, and in everything give thanks, if we want to have a quiet and contented heart. I see His hand so clearly in it all, that I am convinced it is the right thing to do. Praise Him that He is Sovereign, and there is nothing too hard for Him to do.

Hold what God gives you in an open hand, so if He chooses to take it, He can do so without hurting you.

January 9, 1987

It is well into the New Year, and tonight I confess to being discouraged by my mother's continual – with NO letup – complaining and whining, which is finally getting to me. I've never seen such a negative, down right ungrateful attitude in all my life!

Tomorrow, I am going to an Elder's Retreat, where a year ago, my name first came up to them. I hope I will hear something definite. Al is trying to get World Concern to take me on, and today, I found an envelope of papers for them, sent to me back in August of '86. It's mainly about deputation or raising support, and all the time consuming tasks I would be asked to do. My heart tells me – just go to Haiti! Go now! I really can not see how it would be better to go through an organization versus just going on my own. I just don't feel that God leads everyone in the same way. The fact that I am all of these things – old, female, really untrained as a missionary, and with few talents – so why would God lead me in the same way He would a young man planting churches? I just pray that the elders – and myself, will be sensitive to the leading of the Holy Spirit.

I am finished at work – again. My last night, the Lord put me in a room alone with three babies. My little Japanese brother was able to come by for about an hour, and we talked about the things of the Lord. It was good! On New Years Eve, he rushed into the room where I was alone and said he wanted to start the New Year off right by praying with me. I pray that he will continue to grow in the knowledge and wisdom of the Lord, and that the Lord will give him the strength to stand against his family's Buddhist beliefs.

January 10, 1987

I went to Wrightwood to the elder's retreat, and got there about noon.
I took two of the missionary candidate's wives with me. After a nice lunch,
the candidates were asked to give their testimonies, and then tell what they
had done, what ministries they were involved in, and what their hopes for
the future were. When it was my turn, I again said that I wanted to go
back to Haiti to help Pastor Cebien. It was discouraging. Al still hadn't
heard any more from World Concern.

January 20, 1987

My mother and I arrived in Tonopah today about 4:30pm, having left Friendly Valley – for good- about 9:15am. The neighbors next door had invited us to stay with them overnight, since it was after dark by the time the moving van was loaded up that night.

We had two cars, so my trip was a wonderful six hours of music and three of John's tapes on Jude. I am staying at Jeff and Donna's, and my mother at Jim and Pam's.

January 24, 1987

I can't begin to tell how terrible these last three days have been. I just keep praying that the Lord will give my mother a heart of gratitude for all of the good things He has given her here. It's a beautiful house with lots of room, which she says she hates because it's not like the one she left, so that makes it no good at all.

How patient and longsuffering our Heavenly Father is with us, His wayward and self-willed children. How His loving heart must yearn to hear from us words of gratitude and trust. How like the Children of Israel we are with our continual complaining about all that He has NOT given us, and how our yearning for the 'leeks and garlic' of Egypt, must grieve His great heart of love, when what He wants to give us is always SO much better than what He has asked us to give up.

January 30, 1987

The Lord spoke to me twice today, and I am much encouraged. Yesterday, I was slogging through the 'slough of despond,' so to speak. The negative atmosphere in this house was finally drowning me, and I was going under. This morning I sat down to play my little organ, and I found a song by John W. Peterson, and the words were so comforting.

It's Always Darkest Before the Dawn

"Are you discouraged, and are you blue?
Are clouds obscuring the sun from view?
Keep trusting Jesus tho' storms assail,
You have His promise, He will not fail.

He knows your heartache, He understands,
Just put your problem in His great hands;
No trouble meets you, but in His will,
He's not forgotten, He loves you still.

It's always darkest before the dawn,
Don't be discouraged, but carry on;
He'll not forsake you, the sun will break through,
It's always darkest before the dawn.

Then, when I was listening to one of John's tapes, he said this;
". . . . set duty before desire. . . self-discipline to do the difficult task at hand, and set the dream aside until God in His providence makes it possible. A mark of a man in the will of God is that he can have a strong desire burning in his heart, and the measure of that man's commitment to the will of God is – with having that great desire in his heart – how faithful is he to the task at hand?"

I realized that this is my task at hand – getting my mom settled here – while the desire is to be in Haiti. I must be faithful to the task at hand, until God in His providence sends me back to Haiti.

"Thank You my Father for caring so much for me to send me these words to comfort me and set my feet back on the path you have given me".

I tried this morning to get Pastor Cebien on the phone, but got Kathy. I need to know what his itinerary is if he is coming to the States soon. Kathy didn't know, so I'll have to wait until Saturday and call him in Port-au-Prince. Saturday is the anniversary of the Revolution, and I pray that the One who rules all the nations will keep it quiet there.

I am now planning to leave here some time the last week of February. I know that God in His providence will stop me if this is not His will, but I feel I must take a step in some direction to know.

I need to make some plans as – praise the Lord – my mom is doing much better. We had a talk the other night, and I guess she must have spent some time with the Lord, because since then, her attitude has improved wonderfully! She's even cut out a night gown for my grand-daughter's seventh birthday.

I called the storage in Chico, and told them to bring my things to Tonopah, and they should arrive here on the eighteenth of February. I told my mom that I could leave them in storage there if she didn't want them here, but she said it was OK to bring them here.

We had our Tuesday Bible study, and one of the ladies asked me to tell a little about my wanting to return to Haiti, so I did. Several of the women said they would like to hear more, so next Tuesday I will show my slides. I pray they will touch hearts for His glory.

February 12, 1987

Praise the Lord, the light is getting brighter, and at last, I see things beginning to fall into place in God's own timing.

I called Pastor Cebien last Saturday, and he is coming to the States, and will come to Tonopah the first or second week of March. I hadn't heard any more from Grace Church, so I was making plans (in my head) to go back to Haiti with Pastor when he went back. I didn't really feel good about doing it this way, but I just couldn't see anything else happening. In my heart, I didn't want to go with World Concern, but I wanted to do the Lord's will, so since I am not finished in Tonopah, I will wait.

I showed my slides of my three months in Haiti at the Bible study on Tuesday, and the Lord touched hearts. One lady said to me, "I thought everyone lived like we do!" It was certainly an eye opener for some.

Tonight, the phone rang and it was Al Mount. He said that he and Monnie wanted to talk to me. They told me that World Concern was closed to me, (I wanted to shout, "Thank You Lord!") and that I had two options if I still wanted Grace Church behind me. I have never listened more carefully!

Option #1 – I could go with an organization, and let them assign the place of service for me, or,

Option #2 – If I felt that Haiti was definitely God's place for me, that they would be willing for me to go, but – they wanted me to go to language school in Port-au-Prince for a year, or however long it will take for me to learn the language.

Al Warren, in Port, had been asked to investigate Pastor Cebien, so he has been talking to Haitian pastors, and some American missionaries – including Flo. They told me the only positive response Al got was from Flo. When Al Warren pressed them for specific reasons for their negativism, the Haitians would never give him any answer. He also explained that in Haiti there are many jealousy problems. Grace is not too concerned about this report, having met Pastor Cebien themselves. They said they know that Pastor Cebien has a great need, but they don't feel that God has given them Pastor Cebien to care for; but that He has given me to them, so their concern is for my well being. They said they know that if I go down and go right to work, I will be at a great disadvantage and will never learn the language.

At first, my heart was crying, "Oh, no," but the more they said, the better I felt about it. I believe it would be a good compromise. I would be in Haiti. Pastor Cebien usually has a clinic in Port on Saturday, and I could help him there, and get better acquainted with the Warrens, and learn the language. I would only have to stay in Port for as long as it took me to learn, and it might not take me a year.

It really sounds good to me, and Grace Church would be happy, and I would feel so good about that!

"Oh, Father, You are SO good! You are truly the mighty wonderworking God, for whom nothing is too difficult! I thank You, and praise You, and worship You. My heart is filled with the joy of knowing You, and of being Your child. Thy will be done!"

February 14, 1987

Praise the Lord! How exciting to see God at work in our lives! I called Pastor Cebien, to see how he felt about what the elders want me to do, and he agreed! He said that would be fine, and I am so happy that I can now go with Grace Church's blessing! I thank God every day for Grace Church, and for the wonderful group of men who took an old lady seriously, took me by the hand, and told me that if I would submit to their guidance, they would stand by me all the way! I really believe this is God's way to do things, and He has blessed me far over and above all I could ask, or even think. I am SO thankful that I was not forced to choose one over the other, and I thank Him for the guidance of Grace Church, and now we are all in accord just as we should be in Christ. Amen!

February 19, 1987

My furniture was supposed to arrive yesterday, but they called and said it would be tomorrow instead. It snowed again on Wednesday, so it was good it didn't come then.

Today, my world here has come apart. My Kathy surprised us by arriving here about 9:30 last night. My mom was in bed, and I was on my way, when the door bell rang. Donna, my daughter-in-law, had made the trip to Las Vegas, picked her up, and brought her here. Since my stuff had not arrived, we had no bed for her, so Donna took her home with her for the night, as Kathy was very tired.

This morning, I really just had it with my mom. She said, that with my stuff coming, she felt dis-possessed. In other words, she didn't want my things in HER house!

I'm afraid I got upset, and angry, because I had asked her so many times, what did she want me to do? Now, the day it's supposed to arrive, she tells me she doesn't want it here! I could have left it in storage for four years for what it is costing me to bring it here, and she waited until this morning to tell me I was filling her house with my junk. And I got mad! I said some things I shouldn't have – I should have just kept quiet – but I got angry.

This evening, I apologized, and was told, that I didn't really mean it. Then she turned on me and said, "I hate you! I hate you! I hate you!" All I could think was, 'out of the abundance of the heart, the mouth speaks.' Now, I don't know what to do, and poor Kathy, who was trying to get away from stress, walked right into it – big time!

I overheard my mother later, telling Kathy that she wasn't going to help me in Haiti. Doesn't she know that God doesn't need what she doesn't want to give? And it wouldn't really be giving it to me, but to the Lord, and He loves a cheerful giver. My Father owns the cattle on a thousand hills, and He will take care of me. I know He will. I am so sorry that her heart is so full of bitterness. I have no idea why, but she blames me for everything. As long as her attitude is so negative, she will be miserable, and will make everyone around her miserable as well.

I thank God for His forgiveness, and for His keeping power.

February 20, 1987

"Thou knowest not what a day may bring forth."

My poor mother came down stairs this morning with very red eyes, and apologized. I said, she was forgiven, and she asked, if I could forget. I said I'd try, and we would just go on as though it had never happened.

My things came, and in two and a half hours were all over the house. Thank the Lord, it is a very BIG house. It has four bedrooms, and three baths.

After the movers left, Kathy took us to breakfast, and then we came home and started opening boxes. Tonight I sleep in my brass bed again.

I had bought my mother a microwave oven, but yesterday, she told me she was through with me, and she didn't want the microwave. Jim said he would take it back, as I had gotten it at the boy's Sears catalog store, so I boxed it up. Tonight, I noticed it was back on the kitchen counter. It's really difficult to live with a double minded person.

February 27, 1987

I left on Tuesday for California to go to the elder's meeting on Wednesday night. It started at 6:30, and was over at mid-night. I was so thrilled, and humbled, to see my name on Grace Church's budget for two hundred and fifty dollars a month! I didn't know that they would help support me; that was a wonderful surprise.

I was able to get another health insurance policy instead of Blue Cross, for a lot less money. I love the Outreach guys – they have been SO good to me.

"Yet, day by day, the Lord also pours out His steadfast love upon me, and through the night I sing His songs and pray to God who gives me life." Psalm 42:8 LB

I am free now – I can mount up with wings as an eagle. I can fly away! How I praise Him for making me wait upon Him. He is so good and gracious to me.

"Thank You, Lord!!!!!"

March 2, 1987

I'm still waiting for Pastor Cebien to call. I was beginning to wonder if something had happened to him, so this afternoon I called Kathy and Alice. They said that he had only left on Saturday, after his Port-au-Prince clinic, so he's only been in the States for a day, so I'll just have to keep on waiting, I guess. I might as well get used to it; I seem to do a lot of waiting where any Haitians are concerned.

Alice also said she wondered if Grace Church would let her teach me Creole. It sure would be better than in Port, and wouldn't cost as much either, but I doubt if they would agree, since I have already agreed to their plan.

March 7, 1987

I've been thinking that perhaps it would be better if I met Pastor Cebien in Florida, and saved him the trip out here, though I know there are folks here who would like to meet him, as they are very interested in his work. It would save him the money he would spend on a flight out here, plus the time, which I'm sure he can use to a better advantage there. When I asked him on the phone if that might not be a better plan, he said yes, but sounded disappointed. I think he likes my mother's cooking. He once said, "She was a good kook."

March 10, 1987

We finally settled the where and the when. We will meet in Miami on the seventeenth at the Eastern Airline counter, and fly to Port-au-Prince.

March 16, 1987

I arrived in Miami tonight at 9:45. My arms have nearly dropped off carrying my bags. I talked to Pastor Cebien after I bought my tickets in Las Vegas, and he says he will meet me on Wednesday instead of Tuesday. I told him I was going to wring his neck when I saw him. Now, I have a whole day wasted, but maybe I can get my letters written to all the folks on my list.

I really enjoyed being back at Grace Church again and seeing and hearing John again. Saw many good friends, and said 'good-bye' to them. I even got in line to shake John's hand, and told him I was leaving for Haiti. I thank God for so many blessings, especially Grace Church.

Back in Haiti

March 20, 1987

Dr. Al Warren and his gracious wife, Louise, met me at the airport in Port-au-Prince, and I am now sitting on 'my' bed in their home. I praise the Lord for good hearing! The sounds are multi-colored! Everything from Scott Joplin music coming from the piano, (middle Warren son, Brian is playing) to dogs barking, horns honking, people talking, babies crying, and roosters crowing! Isn't this what is known as a cacophony of sound? I love it! I know I'm back in Haiti! However – last night, trying to sleep was another story, especially after the silence of the Nevada desert. I think I probably slept four hours at the most.

This morning, after breakfast, I went with Al to the hospital where he has his dental practice. Again, missionaries do "whatever their hands find to do, as unto the Lord," so today, I was a dental assistant, and helped with two extractions and three root canals. I did the suctioning and fixed the small pick instruments he used for the root canals. I've never seen any of this before, and it was most interesting. We saw one French lady, one Creole, one American, and a German girl from the German Embassy.

We came back to the house and had some cookies and milk about 2pm. Al and Louise are going to a party at the U.S. Ambassador's house tonight where they will probably meet General Namphy, who is running the country at the moment, after another coup, this one by the military.

Sunday, March 22, 1987

I went to church this morning with the Warrens and their three boys, to the English church in Quisqueia where there is a mixed congregation.

After church we went to a music recital, and two of their boys played the piano. The recital lasted for nearly two hours, but it was all worth it just to hear one young Haitian boy play the violin. Spectacular! He really is gifted. I just hope he will be able to use it somehow in this country.

We came home, and had a wonderful Haitian dinner at the Warren's land-lord's house. Last night, Pastor Cebien was invited to dinner, so they finally got to meet him. They were surprised at how young he looked. We had a nice visit with the Warrens while we ate, and then they left to go to a musical. Pastor and I sat at the table and talked about Al Mount's coming visit, and a few other items of business, and then he left.

March 23, 1987

I am going to Cap-Haitian today with Pastor Cebien. He came to the Warren's for me in the big yellow 'Lemozine'. He had picked up a young man at the airport at 4:45, and then came by to get me.

He took us to his house and we waited while he did some things, and then we left again, or so we thought. We stopped next for some chicken, stopped to look for empty bottles, stopped for some napkins, and finally, about 8pm, we left for Cap-Haitien – four of us, plus a lot of baggage. Between Port-au-Prince and Cap-Haitien we stopped for pop, then for candy, then to shut the back doors of the Lemozine, which had popped open, then we stopped to let one man out, and again to fix the windshield wipers. We stopped at a road block, again to shake hands with some men, and visit a bit. We stopped to pick up four more people and their baggage, then to let a girl off, to pick some medicine plants Pastor saw, and finally, after no more stops, we arrived in Cap-Haitien.

We all sang loudly on the way, with Pastor leading; his arm out the window and his hand banging on the side of the machine to keep time, all to the honking of his horn in rhythm. It was unbelievable; lots of fun and good singing. They were all singing in Creole, but the white fellow next to me, and I, sang in English – all at the same time.

At the top of the mountain, we ran into a thick fog, and Pastor said, "he would stay close to the side of the mountain, because if we went off the other side – we would go to Viet Nam!" Very comforting!

The poor kid he had picked up at the airport kept asking me, "What's he stopping for now?"

It was wonderful! We arrived at 1:30 am, and got everybody UP!

March25, 1987

It was wonderful to be back in Flo's house, and to sleep in my room there again. Praise the Lord, He is so good! It's wonderful to see the ones I love everyday. I really don't want to stay in Port-au-Prince, I feel uncomfortable in the Warren's house, like an intruder in their lives.

Flo showed me a letter from Dr. Benson of Medical Ambassadors. In it he warned Pastor Cebien and Flo, "to be careful," and that I "was a very divisive person."

The 'health and prosperity' preacher is still here, and Satan is very busy, and not always through voodoo.

March 26, 1987

We arrived back in Port at 10:30pm after thirteen stops. I counted them this time; there were three to barter and then not buy, three to barter and buy, one to pick up a man, one to let a man out, two to pick plants, two to visit, one house call, and I can't remember the other one.

Al Mount and another man were at the Warren's, so I had to sleep at the neighbor's house, and I hardly even know these people.

March 27, 1987

The afternoon was spent with Al Mount, Al Warren, Bruce, Pastor Cebien, and me, discussing the coming Grace Church team of college age kids.

They finally got around to me, telling me what the elders wanted me to do. I will have to go to language school, though the Haitian-American Institute course is only three months instead of six months, and a hundred and thirty-five dollars, instead of five-hundred and fifty, so again, the Lord is gracious and merciful!

March 28, 1987

After Pastor Cebien's clinic, we left for Cap-Haitien again, so Al Mount and Bruce could check things out for the team that would be coming down. There were thirteen people in the back of the 'Lemonzine' with some luggage, two people on the top, with more luggage, and three of us in the front seat. It was as memorable a trip as all the others have been, and we arrived about 10:30pm in Cap-Haitien. Flo had given me a key, so I got in the house without disturbing her, though when she goes to bed, she takes her hearing aids out of her ears, and says, "Good-bye world!"

March 29, 1987

We went to church in Plaine Du Nord, and Al Mount preached with Pastor Cebien translating from English to Creole as fast as Al preached. Then they went to the first little church Pastor Cebien had built, and Al preached again. After church, Kathy and Alice fixed a wonderful meal for eight of us. They are remarkable, those two!

This evening, we were on our way back to Port, and we stopped at the church where Pastor Dorléon is the preacher, and Al preached again. By the time we reached Pierpine, Pastor Cebien was so tired, he lay down on the floor at Pastor Antoin's, and fell asleep. He just couldn't go anymore, so Al drove the rest of the way to Port, and Pastor Cebien slept in the back. When we got back to the Warren's, we got everybody up again, and rather than get the neighbor up again, (where I was sleeping) I went home with Pastor Cebien and spent the night (what was left of it) on a cot in an upstairs room. I just lay down, and didn't even take my dress off. It was very noisy, but I slept a bit.

March 30, 1987

Pastor Cebien gave me some breakfast, and then we went to the airport to see Al and Bruce off, back to California. They were very happy with their trip, and optimistic about the team's time in the summer. I came back to the Warren's, took a shower and changed my clothes. At 2pm, Pastor Cebien came back and took me to the house where I will be renting a room. It's a beautiful BIG house and I have a room with a bath. There is a shower, but NO hot water.

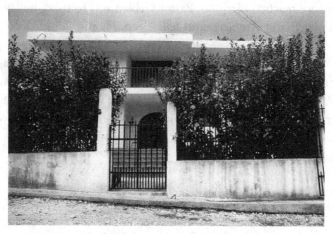

The big house in Petion-Ville

Room and board for $250 a month, not bad! The Lord surely does provide. This house is up the mountain, behind the city of Port-au-Prince in a wealthy district. It's up the same road as the Haiti Baptist Mission, and it is a terrible road; two lane, narrow, and twisting, with the cut side of the mountain on one side, and a steep cliff going down on the other. It is a forty-five minute harrowing drive to the language school, and Pastor Cebien's house is just a few blocks around the corner from the school. He told me that I could stay at his house, but I didn't think that would be a good idea.

He took me to The Haitian American Institute, where I registered for the Creole classes. After driving around in the heat and traffic of Port for three hours, plus practically no sleep the night before, I'm sure that he was wiped out, and needed some rest.

We will be going back to Cap-Haitien again tomorrow, and will come back to Port on Thursday, Lord willing.

I forgot to mention the 'Rah-Rah Band' we ran into just out of one village on the trip here. There must have been fifty to seventy people, some playing strange instruments, some singing, and some doing a shaking type of dance. I didn't know what it was until we were in it, and then we were surrounded.

Pastor Cebien leaned over and quietly said to me, "Roll up the window." They were all around us, banging on the windows and the windshield, and rocking the car. They held on to the car when Pastor stepped on the gas, and kept it from moving. Pastor finally rolled down his window about five inches, and with resonant authority said, "Let go of the machine." They let go, and we were gone! This is all a part of their Mardi Gras. It was a frightening experience – but interesting!

April 2, 1987

We decided to go back to Port in the morning instead of this evening, and I'm glad, as Pastor won't be so exhausted. Our drive to Cap on Saturday was so nice because we had some time to talk. There was only one other lady with us.

April 4, 1987

Our trip back to Port was uneventful, (which was fine with me) and we arrived there about 12:30pm, when he took me back to the Warren's house. About 7pm, he came back by the Warren's on his way back to Cap-Haitien. His wife was with him, plus several other people.

April 7, 1987

I moved to my new house (room) yesterday evening, and got acquainted with the folks that it belongs to, Bob and Carol Caves. It's a very nice place, but I want to buy a desk, and a chair, and especially, a fan! The windows do not open, so the room is very close. I asked the son if there was an extra fan anywhere? He brought me a big fan on a tall stand, and I slept very well. It's much quieter here than it was where the Warrens live. I think it will be a bit difficult to find ways to keep busy here, every day for three months, but it will give me time to study.

Two friends of Pastor Cebien came from California to visit him. I went with him to get them at the airport, and then we went from there to Cap-Haitien.

Pastor had a dream about me, and to him, a dream is the same as reality. The problem is, in this dream, I did something wrong to him, and his whole attitude changed toward me. He has become very distant, and uncommunicative. I have no idea what he thinks I did, so all I can do is wait it out, but it makes life a bit more difficult here.

April 26, 1987

I have been going to language classes, and trying to learn the language. Another boarder here in the house is a missionary named Art. He drives a Daihatsu truck, and works with a Pentecostal group, but he is also going to the Creole classes and I have been able to drive back and forth to the classes with him.

It is a terrifying drive, and his truck must not have any springs at all, as it is very rough and bouncy. The seat seems to slant down, and it is covered with a slick, leather-like material, which I can't seem to stay on. I keep sliding forward, and I have to keep my hands on the dash to stay on the seat; plus, we are going down a pretty steep mountain road. But, it's better than a tap-tap! The classes are difficult for me, but so far, I'm doing ok.

April 29, 1987

Ronnie, our translator in Cap- Haitien, is here in Port, so today we rode from where I live, down the mountain to the city on a 'tap-tap.'

We walked all over Port, and saw lots of things, the beautiful big, white National Palace for one. It's really too bad that this country doesn't have a decent government. Every man who gets the power, steps on all the ones who helped him get there, and then he becomes a greedy, grasping dictator. It doesn't matter if he was a good man before, it happens this way every time there is a change – and these days, it seems to be changing frequently. I laughed at a cartoon in the newspaper the other day. It was a picture of a Haitian man in front of his TV. The newsman was saying, "It's 10pm, do you know who your President is?"

Ronnie and I then rode a 'tap-tap' to an area called Kenskoff, and had dinner in a restaurant there. I had goat, and Ronnie had conch. Then we rode to the school, where I ran into Pastor Cebien, who had my mail. He is still unhappy with me, and I feel very badly about it, but there is nothing I can do, as I really haven't done anything that I can correct.

May 1, 1987

The days here in Port-au-Prince are long and lonely, but the Lord is my constant companion. Praise His Name!

Today, Art told me that he may drop out of language school, and the Caves, (the people who own the house) are leaving in June to go home to the States for awhile. I won't have any way to get to and from class, if Art quits, and I really don't want to spend every day here alone.

Pastor Cebien bought me a car, but it's been in a fix-it shop since he bought it, and I have no idea what the status of it is right now. I haven't talked to Pastor in two weeks, as I have no way to get in touch with him. The Caves have very generously offered to let me drive their little car while they are gone. *"Thank You, Lord!"*

May 30, 1987

It's been a long time since I have written in this, but it's been a rather uneventful time. Last week I made another trip to Cap-Haitien with Pastor Cebien. (Yes, he is talking to me now, though I still don't know what I did.)

He always has so many errands to do before we can leave town. When we got to Pierpine, we stopped, and it was decided that we would stay there for the night with Pastor Antoine and his family. Pastor Cebien had heard that there were road blocks, and people were being stopped, and then robbed, so he didn't want to go on in the dark. There were seven or eight of us traveling in the Lemonzine, and Pastor Antoine put everybody up, though Pastor Cebien slept on the floor, and I think the other passengers slept in the machine, or outside somewhere. Someone there gave up their bed for me, and even brought me a bucket to use for a toilet, so I probably had the best accommodation of anyone. I noticed the inside walls of the rooms were all open about a foot and a half from the ceiling, and you could hear all the conversations going on.

The poor Lemonzine is falling apart. Everything on it is broken. On one trip, Ronnie came back to Cap with Pastor, and he was driving so Pastor could sleep. I'm afraid he was awakened very suddenly when Ronnie put the car in a ditch, and bent the headlights. Now one of them lights up the tops of the trees along the road. They had to take the spotlights off of the roof, and put them down on the front bumper, where they could be used as headlights. I had to drive it from Port to Cap with this arrangement one time, and it was a very tense drive. I hope he got some of it fixed today.

He told me that my car is nearly ready. All it needs is a license sticker, and a battery. I think the battery came, but it's in customs, and I'll have to go and get it out.

I have been driving my landlord's little Mazda Charade back and forth to school, as they told me I could use it while they were gone, and it's been a life saver!

One night, there was a storm, with a lot of rain, and thunder and lightning. When my class was over I began the drive up the mountain to

Pétionville, but when I got to the place where the two lane road began, there were big boulders that had rolled down the hill onto the road. They weren't blocking the way, so I started up in the pouring rain. When I got to the turnoff to the house, it was deep mud, and I was afraid to drive into it. I stayed on the paved road, and drove around up behind the house, where there was an abandoned hotel, and drove under the cover of the admitting area, and got out.

The continuous flashing of lightning was the only light I had. The front entry was open, but it was really spooky walking through this dark empty building with lightning flashing, and thunder crashing, but I felt along the wall and went through and out the back, where there was a big swimming pool, full of rainwater and garbage at the deep end. I walked around the pool, across a field of corn, and then down into the yard of the house, and the back door.

I was soaking wet, but I felt safe at last, and thanked the Lord for being with me.

June 3, 1987

I went with Anne and Leta, two nurses from the Pentecostal Holiness Mission, to their remote clinic in a terrible place called Laroche, or The Rock. It was aptly named as that's all there was there, just rocks, dirt, some scrubby brush, and no water. They must get water from somewhere, but it must be very little. The hills and mountains around were all denuded with no trees at all.

On the way there, yet still in this area, we were asked to stop at a Pastor's house. When we got there, they said there was a sick baby who needed to be seen. We discovered it to be a tiny seven month preemie who died while we were examining him. He couldn't have weighed more than two pounds, yet he had lived for eight days. When I put my stethoscope on his tiny boney chest, I heard only an occasional gasp, and a heart rate of 60, which in a baby that size is equivalent to cardiac arrest. He was ice cold to touch, and his clothing, such as it was – mostly strips of cloth and a tiny shirt and hat – was cold and damp. His dark eyes were open and unblinking, and his tiny hands and feet scarcely moved.

Leta tried spooning some Pedialyte into his mouth, but it was useless. Poor tiny mite, yet fortunate in a way, to be spared a life of struggle in such a poor place. We did what we could, and went on.

At a brush arbor church, we set up our tables with medicines and equipment. Anne and I diagnosed, and Leta and Rick, (Art's son who was visiting) passed out the medicines. Kirby, a fellow who has just moved into a room at the house, until his wife arrives in July, helped the Pastor write names on the prescription slips and passed out numbers.

Art helped keep order, and also passed out medicines. It was really a good thing we had the men with us as it would have been impossible to keep any order at all. These folks have NO medical help, NO school, and only just recently got this brush arbor church.

They were frantic for help, and all wanted to be seen. We saw 140 people, and ran out of some medicines, mainly worm medicine, as everyone had some kind of worms.

We also saw a lot of really bad skin problems, which was no surprise in such a dirty, dusty area, with such a limited water supply. For many of them, we couldn't do much. We gave out a lot of soap, but with so little water, it would be only a temporary fix at best. Several children had dirt literally caked on their faces. It really made me feel helpless, and very sad, to see them living like this.

The wind was blowing, and I frequently got a face full of dust and dirt. When we ran out of medicines and had to quit, there was a near riot. There were still quite a few who hadn't been seen, and with no hope of anyone helping them again for who knows how long, maybe a month or more, they were desperate!

I was really glad to leave, but I kept thinking of how much the Lord has given to us. I was thankful that I could leave, and in a car with air-conditioning! I could get out of the rocks and dirt, and go back to a clean place to eat good food, to sleep in a clean bed, and best of all – where there was water to take a bath and wash my hair; while they had no other place to go except that place of rocks and dirt. They probably were wondering how they were going to use the soap we had given them – with so little water.

They are so poor, and my heart aches for them. How the great heart of God must weep over the misery of these poor people, for He truly loves the poor, and their plight concerns Him.

June 11, 1987

It's so strange to think that when my son Jeff was born in 1950, there was a little six year old Haitian boy named Cebien (it is good) who was learning herbal medicine from his grandmother, and because of a faithful missionary, or pastor, that little boy grew up to be one of God's choice laborers in Haiti.

In the 1970's two young American girls were searching for God's place for them, and heard the young man from Haiti. God gave them a love for him, and when he asked them to come and work with him in Haiti, they said yes. Then a year ago, my life also became entwined for the Lord with this man, Pastor Cebien, and Kathy and Alice, the two girls. It will never be the same again, for which I thank and praise the Lord!

I have been chauffeuring Pastor all over Port-au-Prince for three days. His feeding program for his schools is killing him. He feeds every child in his many schools, one hot meal a day, and it takes a lot of food, mostly rice and beans, but he is having a hard time finding it, and then sometimes it gets stolen on the way to the schools. It takes nearly all of his time and money.

Everyone in the house here is gone. Carol left on the first and the fellows are in Lascahobas for a week with a team of twenty-six teenagers. I gave Nana, the house maid here, the day off yesterday and today, and it's been kind of nice with no one around. Nana was sneezing all over the place and had a runny nose, so I really didn't need her around, and she needed to rest.

My Creole classes are a disaster. The teacher is going too fast for me now, and I just can't keep up. I think what would help me now is a tutor.

June 22, 1987

The team of young people is arriving from Grace Church today in Port-au-Prince, but there is a general strike on, and no one is allowed on the streets. They've warned that any cars out will be smashed and burned.

Pastor Cebien plans to go to the airport tonight anyway to pick them up, but I think I will stay here as I don't want anything to happen to the landlord's car. Al Warren has been driving around this morning – I don't really know why – but he seems to think everything is OK.

After I wrote the entry of June 11, Pastor Cebien went to Cap-Haitien on a tap-tap with 96 bags of milk for his schools and his orphanage. Before they got to Pierpine they came to a roadblock, and thieves stole all 96 bags of the milk. He said they had rocks and machetes, so there was nothing he could do. That's another big loss for him. My car is probably another loss for him. It's been four or five months since it was purchased, and it's still not ready.

Pastor Cebien was able to get to the airport with no problem. He picked up the team of teens from Grace Church and brought them all to my place here for some chicken, and then took them all back to his house to stay until we can get through to Cap-Haitien.

I learned something else about Pastor Cebien that was interesting. He said that he was born in England, and was brought to Haiti by his mother when he was only four years old. He must have been speaking English, and Creole, and then had to re-learn English again much later. He says he still has family in England. This might mean that he is really a citizen of England.

June 27, 1987

The team has had a busy week, but a lot of it has been spent waiting for Pastor Cebien. They are getting a big dose of time value in the Haitian culture.

Poor Pastor Cebien has had so many problems – some of them with the Lemonzine. I came down the mountain early this morning to Pastor's house to take the kids to the Warren's for breakfast. My first problem was getting the key to the Lemonzine. (I don't think that Pastor was up yet.) Then, I couldn't get it started, and he had to get up, come and get it started for me. It was very hard to steer as one front tire was nearly flat.

As we went by the Holiday Inn right in the middle of town, there was a crowd around a car and under the car was a person that had been hit, I guess. It was awful, and I hurried to get out of town and away from the scene. (I wonder if they killed the driver of the car that caused the problem, because that's what they do here.)

We made it to the Warren's, and had a nice breakfast, and visit with Al. When we were ready to leave, I had gotten the Lemonzine so close to the wall, I couldn't get it away from it, and Al had to come and jockey it out for me. We put some air in the tire, and made it back to Pastor Cebien's house.

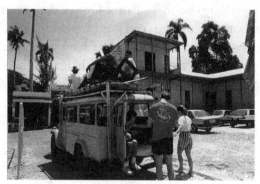

The Lemonzine

I helped him in the clinic, and we were through by 1pm, when he left to do something. The team all waited for him until 5pm, when he finally came back, and took the kids to the beach on Cacique Island.

One of the girls was on another kid's shoulders in the water, and dove off, not realizing there was coral there, and scraped her pretty face on it. So, now we have three in pain. One boy came with a bad back, and now it's worse, another has a hurt foot, and now this poor girl.

I have to say that their attitude is exceptional, and their parents and Grace Church would be very proud of them. They are really being stretched, and sometimes it can be painful.

I seem to be always running between them and Pastor Cebien, trying to smooth out the path for all of them, but they are a super nice bunch of kids.

Oh, yes, on the way back to Pastor's home, the drive shaft nearly fell out in the street. We were a good 45 minutes looking for the two bolts to put back in it so we could get back home.

June 29, 1987

Another strike today, so we were unable to do anything. The strike last Monday was called by a labor union, but this one today was across the board. It seems that General Namphy likes the power he has now, and the people are protesting – afraid that they will end up with another dictator like Duvalier. It's so good to know that our God is sovereign, and is still in control of the nations of this world. He sets up and puts down those whom He wills.

I had been hoping that we would be going to Cap-Haitien, but I doubt we will if the strike continues. I should get to Flo's house as she is gone, and she expected me to be there this week. The mail comes again tomorrow, and I still don't have last weeks mail yet.

I think my car is ready now – at least I saw it in Pastor's driveway yesterday. Speaking of yesterday – I was in front of Pastor Cebien's house, talking with two other pastors. The Lemonzine was parked in the front, headed down hill in front of the driveway, as Pastor had been working on the battery, because the lights wouldn't work.

It had been sitting there for about 15 minutes, with the driver's door open. Suddenly, it just started to roll down the street all by itself! Both pastors jumped, and one jumped in and stepped on the brake. (The emergency brake doesn't work) If we hadn't been standing right there, it would have rolled down the street, and ended up in the fish market. That machine is really something! It has its own personality.

July 1, 1987

The strike has carried over through Tuesday, and now Wednesday has been declared a free day. In other words, their war just stops for a day, so people can go to the stores and stock up again. The protest against General Namphy goes on. He spoke on TV last night, but said nothing of any importance.

About 10am, I went to pastor Cebien's house with my belongings, and as usual, he was gone. The team was all packed to go to Cap-Haitien, and were waiting for him. My car was supposed to be ready, but they were working on it again.

Yesterday another team came in from Teen Missions to work with him, and he had gone to town to try to arrange transportation for 33 kids to Cap-Haitien, and I think he was also arranging for his family (they had come back) to leave again for the States.

I took him to see about my car – not ready – and driving thru the city, I had to turn around once because of a road block. There were burned buses, cars, and trucks in the streets. One of the main streets was absolutely black from so much stuff being burned there, and my hands and face were also black after I drove through it.

Finally, about 4:15pm, we were ready to leave. I was going to drive my borrowed car to the Warren's, and Pastor Cebien was going to pick me up there. He had a Haitian lady, and all the team kids in the Lemonzine, and there really was no room for me. When I could see that it was going to take me too long to get to the Warren's, I turned around, and met him coming up the hill. I told him to forget about taking me, and just to go on, it was too dangerous to delay any longer, and I wanted him to get those kids to a safer place as soon as he could. I would be OK in the house where I was. The other team of kids was waiting for him just out of town.

So, here I am   back at the Cave's house on Laboule Drive, when I wanted so much to get to Cap. It's so disappointing, but I know Who is in control – both of the Nations, and also my small self. Praise the Lord!

Tomorrow will be a very bad day I'm sure, as the people become increasingly angry with the government, which is General Namphy at the moment. Already ten civilians have died in clashes with soldiers, and scores have been hurt. Not even an ambulance could get through on the streets. I just hope that Gonaives will not give Pastor Cebien any problem. It seems that it's always worse there, and frequently, it's the town where the trouble starts.

July 2, 1987

Namphy is still refusing to yield. Now, a Catholic Bishop has gotten into the act, and is telling the people not to be satisfied with him yielding, but to force him out totally. There was a lot of violence today, especially in the Carrefour area, where one person was killed and several injured. I heard of one death in Cap-Haitien. A lot of vehicles and tires have been burned in the streets.

There was a demonstration at the Haiti Baptist Mission, and they were forced to close their restaurant and shop, and there were also several road blocks between here and the Mission. Art learns a lot on his C.B. radio, and we saw some pictures of Carrefour on the TV. Thank the Lord, I am quite safe here, at the house, where He has seen fit to keep me. Al Warren left for the States today. I guess he's coming back, but he may not..

July 5, 1987

I finally got to Cap-Haitien in my car. Pastor Cebien had come back to Port, so he drove with me. I was very glad that he was with me, as this car is not very dependable. We went through road block after road block; all open, but still there.

We saw all the road blocks that Pastor Cebien had to go through with the kids, only then it was dark, and there was fire to pass through with all those kids. It was a harrowing experience, one they will never forget. They had to pass through crowds of people with clubs and machetes, who didn't want to let them pass. Pastor said they were stopped four times. It was 4:30 in the morning when they finally got to Morne Rouge, and could feel safe. Twelve hours of fear for all those kids, and for Pastor, too. I was glad I hadn't gone, but then, I also felt like I had been done out of a real adventure!

I finally got to Flo's only to find that Medical Ambassadors had sent a Doctor down, without telling me, and he was now living in the house while Flo was gone! He met me at the door, with a big, "Hi, I'm Doctor Mike!" I was shocked! He is a big, handsome, thirty year old Irishman, unmarried, at the moment, but he's had three, and – this I really can NOT believe, he is – not a Christian! Sent here by a mission board!

Again, the twists and turns of my life are something else! I hope he sees me as a very old and undesirable female, and stays out of my way! He is pleasant, but very worldly; drinking, smoking cigars, and going to the porno movies in town; taking some of the young Haitian boys with him. Really bad example. I can not imagine why they sent him down here, especially while Flo is away, and they know I'm here alone.

July 6, 1987

One of the Haitian boys, Paul, who was always at the airport, and now hangs out with Dr. Mike, said to me, "Why are you sad? When you were here before, you were happy."

A very astute observation, indeed! I didn't feel that I was sad, but I guess I'm just not 'happy' in the way I was then. I'm certainly not unhappy, but he saw some kind of difference that I really was not aware of.

The Pastor's Conference is in session here now, but I have nothing to do in it. Pastor Cebien is so busy, running in all directions at once, and he is exhausted. He has no time to talk to me about anything, but today I managed to get ten minutes, because I wanted to talk to him about what I should do about Dr. Mike. I can't believe that Dr. Benson would actually send someone who is not even a Christian to represent Christ. There is no way that he can represent Christ. He is a real party boy, and a very bad example for some of the weaker young people here, though they think he's wonderful. He even gives them drinks and cigarettes.

It's putting both Pastor Cebien and me in a very bad position. Here I am, living in the same house with him, and Pastor Cebien represents Medical Ambassadors, and so does this man – it's got to be confusing to those who are watching our lives, and lumping us all together. I really don't know what to do. Pastor Cebien doesn't seem to be concerned, and that confuses me, and I really have no other place to go.

The roof is still not on my part of the clinic, so I don't have much to do, and I just don't know what to do right now. Pastor Cebien keeps saying that I must make up my own mind, but it would really be nice to have a bit of input from him. I feel like I am walking in the dark, but God is not the author of confusion.

July 8, 1987

Tonight was the last night of the Pastor's Conference, and I wouldn't have missed it for anything. Pastor Cebien was priceless! He really felt good, and was playing his accordion so well, and really enjoying it. His face tells everything that is in his heart, and tonight was reflected the joy of the Lord. What a precious man. He's certainly not perfect, but he comes pretty close. I love watching him preach and sing.

Speaking of singing – I can't believe it, but Pastor Cebien asked me to sing a duet with him tonight for the whole church! I figured every body else gets up and sings, and some of them are pretty terrible, but no one seems to mind, so I thought they won't mind it if I'm terrible, too. I just didn't want to embarrass Pastor Cebien.

You might know – the lights went off just before we were supposed to sing, so I went up to the platform with my flashlight and my Creole songbook. It was probably better that the lights were out – I couldn't see anyone out there. I think one of the team taped it, and someone took a picture, because a flash went off in my face.

The guest preacher for the last service of the Pastor's Conference was a young man from Grace Church, and he really got the works tonight. The lights went on and off, and then the rain started. It poured, and on the tin roof of the church it was so loud, we couldn't hear him at all. It finally slowed down, and then stopped.

The service was over about 11pm, and Pastor was going to take me and one of the team members home as she was sick, and then the men and Pastor Cebien were going to have some Haitian coffee together. Well, one of the Pastors had gone home with the key to the Lemonzine in his pocket, so there we sat, all ready to go, when Pastor Cebien walked up and said, "Oh. Miss Pat, we have a problem." We had to go across the street to another missionary's house, and she was sweet enough to take us home.

The next morning, Pastor Cebien was helping all the pastors work on his orphanage roof. He was so tired, he went to sleep on the roof. Poor man! He needs someone to take care of him, and though Kathy and Alice try, he doesn't really cooperate! He only knows how to give.

July 12, 1987

Today the team went to a remote clinic with Pastor Cebien and I, that is, all of the team but two of the girls who were sick, and they are staying at Flo's, much to Dr. Mike's disgust. The rest of the team stays at Morne Rouge with Pastor Cebien. When Pastor said Belle Aire, I thought it was the place that we had been to for clinics with Dorléon, but I learned too late that it wasn't.

We had to begin our walk sooner than when we were here before, as the road was too badly washed out to drive the Lemonzine over it.

When we got to the little waterfall, I thought we were almost there. Then we made a sharp right turn, and really started climbing. It was again as far as we had already come, and it went up at a very steep climb! I wasn't sure I was going to make it, but I did, and I also made it back, thanks to the strength the Lord gave me. It was a six mile round trip.

Just before I got to the village and crossed the last river, I heard Pastor yelling, "Yea! Miss Pat made it!" Then, I had to wade across the river, and when I got to where everybody was, I asked Pastor Cebien, "Uh, when does the helicopter come to pick us up and take us back?" He just laughed at me.

I don't know if Pastor is going to have his clinic this week or not. The roof on my part of the clinic is still not on, so here I sit.

How easy it is to fall back and how hard to keep your eyes on the goal, and climb. I learned that yesterday! Now, it impresses me spiritually.

July 20, 1987

I haven't seen much of Pastor Cebien since he went to Port-au-Prince on Thursday, and came back early Sunday morning.

Yesterday evening in English Church, I read these wonderful verses in Isaiah 43:1-3 "But now, the Lord who created you. . . says, "Don't be afraid for I have ransomed you, I have called you by my name, you are mine. When you go through deep waters and great trouble, I will be with you. When you go through rivers of difficulty, you will not drown. When you walk through the fire of oppression, you will not be burned up – the flames will not consume you." LB

Then in chapter 42:16 of Isaiah it says, "He will make the darkness bright before them and smooth and straighten out the road ahead. He will not forsake them." LB

It doesn't say we will not have problems, but rather the opposite – we will have – deep waters, great troubles, rivers of difficulty, and fire through which we will have to walk. But He also says, "I will be with you. You won't drown, and you won't be burned!" Praise the Lord!

Dr. Mike is really a problem! He is drinking, smoking cigars, swearing, and going to porno movies. He is foul mouthed, and insists on walking around in his underwear! All of this is very hard for me to deal with. He is much more interested in voodoo than in Scripture, and one night, he came to my bedroom door drunk, very maudlin, telling me he was lonesome. I was glad I could lock the screen, and I told him that I was NOT lonesome, and to go back to his own room. Thank the Lord, He went.

Lord willing, Flo will be home tomorrow, and then she can deal with this problem. I hope she will call Dr. Benson, but I don't know. The really sad thing is that he thinks he's a Christian. Someone has given him a false assurance that since he belongs to a specific church, he is on his way to Heaven. Now he is merrily going down the broad road to destruction, thinking he is on his way to Heaven. I don't know what Medical Ambassadors was thinking when they sent him here. Maybe Dr. Benson thought I would leave if he was here, and Flo wasn't. Maybe I should have.

July 28, 1987

Flo came home last Tuesday, and was very upset by what she found. She finally went and called Dr. Benson yesterday, and then told Mike he had 24 hours to leave the house. Poor guy, I can't help but feel kind of sorry for him; he takes his lumps well. Today, he left, and as I drove him to a friend's house, (where he said he would stay with a witchdoctor) I told him his life would only get worse and worse, until he admits that he is a sinner, at the end of his own resources, and turns his life over to Christ. He is confused and hurting, I know, and I pray that he will turn to Christ. There is NO other way.

Pastor Cebien came today after being gone for a week. He's taking the Teen Missions team back to Port-au-Prince so they can return home tomorrow. He said that next week will be bad trouble all over Haiti, and now it's the Americans who are being blamed for helping General Namphy. Maybe Heaven is nearer than we think. Praise the Lord!

August 2, 1987

Port-au-Prince has been a regular war for several weeks now. Many people have been killed, their bodies were loaded on a truck, and they were taken out and buried. Here in Cap-Haitien, it has been quiet. No road blocks or problems of any kind.

Beginning tomorrow, they have called for a general strike in the whole country, so Flo and I have stocked up on food and other supplies, so we shouldn't have to go out to the store for quite a while. I hear the drums every night, but that may, or may not, mean anything.

Doctor Mike is now living at Hotel Paradise, just up the street. He said he killed two tarantulas at his friend's house, so he moved. Also, he said it was too noisy being right behind the Esso gas station. When Mike called Dr. Benson, he was told not to leave Haiti, much to Flo's disgust.

Pastor Cebien came by tonight and told us that he had gotten all the team kids out of the country, so he won't have to worry about their safety anymore. I hope I hear from some of my Grace team kids, they were such a sweet bunch of young people. They came to tell me 'Good-bye' the night before they left for Port, and when I went to the door, they all said, "We love you, Miss Pat". They had made a banner that said the same thing, and I have it on the wall in my room now. We had a 'prayer-party', and it was very sweet.

August 6, 1987

I can't believe how the time is going by. Today was the second time I went and worked in Diana's clinic. I went last Thursday and helped with diagnosing. Today I was the lab technician, and ICU nurse. I pricked fingers, spun hematocrits and total proteins; I gave oral rehydration solution, and even put a stool specimen under the microscope and found – ugh – a round worm. That took me awhile as I didn't really know what I was doing.

I also spent about 45 minutes opening an abscess on the scalp of a two year old. Since we have no gloves to wear I'm afraid I did think about AIDS a couple of times in all of this, but then there were so many other terrible things, like typhoid, malaria, and staph infections, that I really didn't spend much time dwelling on AIDS. Some of our patients probably do have it, but we have no way to know.

Several really ill kids today, two of whom, Diana sent to Limbé. Last Thursday, they made a video during the clinic, and I think I was in it. Diana's husband, John, is leaving for the States tomorrow, and he will be showing it in nine churches in the south.

In the town of Jérémie, there is a man whose whole family was wiped out by Papa Doc Duvalier. He has come back to Haiti from the States, raised his own personal army, and is out for revenge. He's going to start his own war, and then we'll have separate little wars everywhere.

In Jean-Rabel in the north of Haiti, the communists have been causing great problems, and many people have been killed. The Catholic Church there has split over it, and half have elected to go with the communists. It doesn't seem that any of this has anything to do with the real political situation of the President in Port-au-Prince, but there are a lot of undertones that we are not aware of. We have been told that next week will be a bad one, but we were told that last week too, and it was very normal, with no problems here in Cap-Haitien, so we never know what to believe.

On Monday, as I was taking three other white missionaries into town, we started through the police gates, (there's no other way into the town) and we were stopped by soldiers. One walked over to the car, after motioning me to stop, opened my door, and said, "Déscend!" (get out)

I said, "Déscend?" and stayed where I was, playing dumb, though I did understand that word, I didn't want to get out. He then looked in my purse, the glove compartment, the back seat, under the seats, and though I don't know what he was hoping to find, I guess he was satisfied that we didn't have it, whatever it was, and said we could go. That was my first scare of the day.

Later that day, I got into the shower, and as I pulled the curtain closed, a big frog went sailing over my shoulder from somewhere behind me, and landed on the wall, just in front of my face with a big splat! Well, I very quickly got out, and let him have it.

I put my clothes back on, and went out to find something to catch him with. I found a plastic bowl, but every time I tried to put it over him, he jumped in another direction. During the process of chasing him around the shower, he took a big jump, and landed on me!

That's when I went for reinforcements. I tried Ma'Louie first, but, like most Haitians, she was more afraid of the frog than I was. Next, I went next door to get Sandy and he came with a big machete, but only succeeded in chasing it into the motor part of the washing machine. So, next came Raoul, the yard man, with a big can of bug spray and finally, the poor thing crawled out of the washer and was put out of it's misery - and I finally got my shower!

After dinner, we had a sudden thunder shower, with a most impressive display of lightning, and very loud claps of thunder. When the wind blew several doors shut with big bangs, it scared Nikki, Flo's cat, and she streaked out the front door, leaped over the dog, and was gone. I was trying to see where she went, when lightning struck the porch rail in front of my face. The sound, and the brightness of it were spectacular and frightening. The dog took off one way, and Nikki, who had come back, went the other – right out into the pouring rain and mud! I thought we probably wouldn't see her again until the next day, but she found some dry place where she felt safe, and came back when it was over.

Then – still later – I was in my room, listening to a tape, when out of the corner of my eye, I saw something moving on the floor out in the hall. My first thought was 'mouse' as that was about how big it was. Then – I saw what it really was. It was a mammoth mouse- size beetle! I grabbed the fly swatter, and gave it a few good whacks, and flipped it under the table. The next day, it was gone! Tonight – here it is again – slightly the worse for the whacks, but still navigating. Boy! Are they hard to kill. I killed it again, only this time, I think it will stay dead!

August 23, 1987

It's been awhile since I have written in here, and several things have happened. I'm continuing to work in Diana's clinic on Tuesday and Thursday, and now I've progressed to writing prescriptions, as well as diagnosing. Some of these kids are not far from death, and it takes several hours of slowly giving them oral rehydration solution before they begin to come back. Dehydration and malnutrition are the two 'biggies' here. There was a three year old that weighed fifteen pounds, a fourteen month old that weighed fourteen pounds, and a two month old that weighed five pounds; one three year old with really bad kwashiorkor, lots of kids with measles, malaria, typhoid, TB, and on and on. All compounded by malnutrition and worms. It's six to nine hours of continuous sweating, and all to the accompaniment of non-stop loud crying, sometimes so loud I can't hear what the mother, who is sitting right in front of me, is saying.

On Wednesday, I'll go with Flo to Belle Hotesse for a remote clinic, where we see about one hundred people. Pastor Maizamo will go with us, and since he's been in Flo's Village Health Worker's class, he can also diagnose.. He is a very sweet young Haitian man who really loves the Lord.

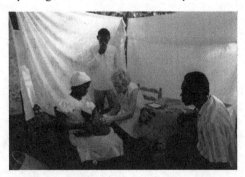

Pastor Maizamo on the right and I in his clinic

Pastor Cebien had put him in a church with an older pastor, and there were some problems. Pastor Cebien took him out of the church and told him to wait, and he would give him another church. He's been waiting for a long time now, and he's found a church building right where he lives, and it's for sale for fifteen hundred dollars. He came to Flo and me to ask if we could give him the money to buy it. We worked out a plan, and gave him five hundred dollars for a down payment, and then we'll give him a hundred dollars a month to make his payments. His heart and motives are right, and he really wants to preach.

Sandy's house next door was broken into one night, and the dog was barking and barking. It was 3:30 in the morning, and I couldn't see who, or what he was barking at, because they were around on the other side of the house. (Once, when the dog was barking at night, it was because a great big pig sauntered through our front yard in the middle of the night, and made the dog go nuts.)

Meg and Wilber, another couple who are missionaries, were staying next door in Sandy's house while he was in Canada, but Wilber was gone at this time, so Meg was alone. I heard her call me from a window, and she said that someone was breaking into the house, and there was a knife cutting the screen in the window. She was afraid because they weren't stopping, even though they knew she was there and was awake.

She took the TV, and came to our house. Now, there is a guard there at night. Praise God for His safekeeping!

September 1, 1987

I worked in the clinic today, and had a baby try to die on me. It was a small three week old girl, whom the father had brought in, because the mother was also sick.

The baby probably had pneumonia. Her lungs were full, her color was cyanotic, and her respiratory rate was irregular, with periods of apnea.

I started giving her some oral rehydration solution with a syringe, and she took it very well. After about an hour and a half, I mixed up some formula, and was showing the dad how to feed her. I was hoping to send her home, and have the dad bring both the mom and baby back tomorrow.

As I watched, I noticed that she had stopped breathing, so I flipped her foot, and got no response. When the dad had first brought her in and laid her down for me to examine, she was unresponsive, and floppy. When I gave her an injection of penicillin, I got very little response with only a weak cry.

When I saw that she had quit breathing, and I had no response to a flipped foot, I listened for a heart beat, and got a heart rate of about sixty. It should have been 120-140 at least.

I took her from the dad, went through the consulting room, saying, "Diana, this baby is dying!" I laid her on the examining table, put my hands around her chest, and started CPR with my two thumbs. I said, "Somebody has to breath for this baby, I have a cold!" Diana's husband, John said, "I'll do it, but you'll have to tell me how!"

I very quickly told him, and after he had given her about four puffs, she gasped, and then began to breathe on her own again. Her heart rate came up to 140, and she began to pink up, and was now pinker than she had been in all the time she had been there.

As usual, the crowd was there to watch the drama, and while we worked on the baby, you could have heard a pin drop.

When she started to breathe again, Diana shouted, "Praise God!" and everyone there began to shout, talk, and laugh. We were all so relieved!

I sent someone to get the father, and as he came around the corner, he was wiping the tears from his eyes; he had been crying. He thought he

231

had lost his baby girl, but then he smiled and couldn't stop smiling when he saw that she was alive.

Now, in the States, that baby would have been put on a ventilator, been given IV's with antibiotics, and IV feedings, monitors, and the whole nine yards, but since this is Haiti – she was put on the back of her father's motor bike, and taken to the city hospital, where she may die anyway.

Sometimes, what we do here seems like an exercise in futility. Then I remember, that all God asks, is that we be found faithful in what it is that He has asked us to do. Sometimes, I feel that I am being asked to do the impossible, but then I remember that the impossible is His business, not mine. Mine is to be obedient to His word, and live it out every day.

September 6 note: I found out that this baby did well, and went home! Praise the Lord – He still is in the business of doing the impossible! AMEN! Praise the Lord!

September 2, 1987

Kathy and Alice and I went to another missionary's house tonight for dinner, but Flo didn't want to go.

After dinner, while we were playing Bible Trivia, we had a good strong earthquake, probably a 3 or 4 on the Richter scale, lasting about 30 seconds. It's the first one I've felt in Haiti.

The three year old that I mentioned on August 23rd, came back in to the clinic a week later, and was nearly dead. She had intractable diarrhea, and was severely dehydrated. I started an IV in her foot, and it ran until about a half a liter had gone in, over about ten hours. Her abdomen was as hard as a rock. She died three days later at another nurse's house. Diana thinks she had a bowl perforation.

Poor baby, she's with the One who loves her most, now and forever! Praise the Lord for the hope we have in Christ Jesus! Amen!

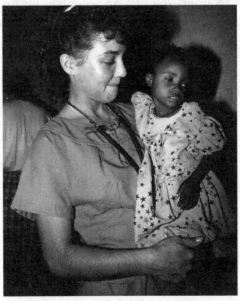

Darlynn and a very sick child

September 6, 1987

Flo and I went to Pastor Maizamo's church this morning to see how he was doing. We got there while he was teaching Sunday school. He was drilling the kids on a Bible verse, and they did it over and over. Those kids will never forget it.

The church building is made of small woven sticks, dirt floor, and tin roof. During the sermon, a rooster strolled through, lizards ran all over the rafters, and the kids were doing what kids do everywhere when they are bored – wriggle and squirm!

Pastor Maizamo is a very nice young man, who really loves the Lord. His sermon was good, at least what I could understand of it. He was wearing a suit and tie, as all Haitian pastors do – out of respect for the Lord and the church – but it was so hot, that he was wiping the sweat off of his face every two minutes.

I must see about getting him an accordion for his church. They are very good at teaching themselves how to play an instrument if they can get one.

September 10, 1987

Tonight was the graduation of Flo's Village Health Workers Class. It is supposed to be a six month course, teaching them basic health principles, like boiling all water, where to place a latrine, etc. They are also taught most of the signs and symptoms of the most common diseases here, and what medicines to give for each. When they finish, they are supposed to go back to their own village, and teach them all these things they have learned, and they can have clinics with medicines that Flo has taught them to give, and provides for them. It's a very good concept, and should prevent a lot of health problems in the future.

Because of the political problems, and the unrest in the country, the class was much longer than six months because there were so many days that Flo couldn't have her class, due to the unrest in the country.

So- tonight was the big finale, their Graduation and giving out of certificates. The church at Morne Rouge was festooned with hanging toilet paper chains of several pastel colors, and there were potted plants across the front of the big church. It looked very festive, and every one was so excited.

We prayed for electricity, but showed our lack of faith by asking Don Davis to stand by with his generator. It began very well, at about 7:30, instead of the 7:00pm announced on the program, but for Haiti – that's not bad!

Pastor Livingston gave the opening prayer, then a Welcome by Flo, translated into Creole by Kathy. Next, six girls got up and sang, after which, Flo introduced the guest speaker, Dr. Jocelyn – a Haitian dentist, trained in the U.S., and he is also a graduate of a law school here in Haiti. He is a very nice man, and a Christian. From what I could understand, it was a good message, and then – the lights went out! Total darkness! A few flashlights popped on here and there, and then after a few minutes – Don's generator started up.

Now, we could see Dr. Jo, but we couldn't hear him. We had lights, but the generator was so loud, we could see his mouth moving, but we had no idea what he was saying, as we couldn't hear him at all.

The generator would falter, the lights would dim and then go off, then up would come the noise again, and on would come the lights! This happened about five or six times, then off went the generator, and – on came the lights! Praise the Lord! Only now, Dr. Jo was finished with his message. Poor man, he deserved a medal!

There followed more singing by the girls, and then, Flo and Kathy began the handing out of the certificates.

Kathy and Alice's dog, Pepsi, thought he was graduating too, so he was up there on the platform, walking around, stretching with his rear end up in the air –and aimed at the audience. Then he sat down, yawned, and then lay down, so those coming for diplomas had to walk around him. It was really funny! Flo said she should have made a certificate for him, since he's been to all the classes. (He also goes to church every Sunday.)

It was a very nice graduation, and the students were all proud of their accomplishment. Flo is glad it is finished, but there are already those who want to sign up for the next class!

September 19, 1987

Thursday night, the dogs barked and barked, but we never saw anything, or heard anyone. Friday morning, as I was feeding our dogs, I noticed something strange. The screen over the cement louvered window of the medicine room was torn, and there were a few empty pill bottles sitting on the foundation ledge of the house. Then, as I walked around, I noticed the other window in the medicine room had a big hole in it, and things were scattered on the walk. Someone had torn the screens, reached in, and taken everything within reach, which fortunately, wasn't much. Mostly Aspirin.

It's getting worse and worse here. You almost hate to see the sun go down, because that's when the thieves come out.

Right now, the dog is barking and growling all around the house. I'm glad Sandy is home because when the dogs bark, he always goes out to see what it might be. On one of his trips around our two houses, I heard a stick banging on our metal back door, and my thought was, *"He certainly is a most brazen thief!"*

It was Sandy killing a tarantula as big as his hand, that was crawling up the door. I wish that people here wouldn't kill everything they see. Flo killed a small tarantula today, and Raoul killed a small green snake. These creatures are basically harmless, (though that tarantula was sure big!) but they only do what God created them to do, which is more than I can say for mankind.

We had a good clinic on Friday. After the clinic, Joyce (another American nurse) and Flo brought to our house a two year old boy who had fallen into the family cooking fire. The whole left side of his body had first and second degree burns, including his left ear which was gone. Unfortunately, this happens a lot here.

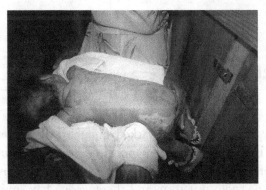

Baby with burns

They put him in Flo's bath tub to soak off some cotton he had stuck to him, and then Joyce took him home with her. Tonight, she brought him back, and now he has a high fever. He managed for seven days in the filth he lives in, to NOT get an infection, and then when we bring him to our clean environment – he gets sick!

I wondered about the water they soaked him in. It comes from the cistern, and we don't drink it, yet this child with open skin areas was put into it, and they put him into it again tonight. Now they're treating him with penicillin. I also wondered about the Silvadene cream which was being put on the open areas of his skin; it was very old, and had been opened. Time will tell.

Later note: This little boy has healed up remarkably well, with minimal scarring, and his skin is even re-pigmenting. Praise the Lord!

September 20, 1987

Our thief returned last night, and cleverly worked all of Flo's aspirin off of the white cabinet, onto the metal shelves where he could get it with his hands through the torn screen. On Thursday, the last of the aspirin Flo had, was packed, and Richard, (the Begger) brought her nineteen thousand more the next day. God's timing is perfect! We had thought the thief had gotten all of it, but some had fallen down behind the cabinet. Seven bottles to be exact, and when she told Richard, he said he would send her ten thousand more!

The thief also broke our faucet by the cistern. He was trying to use it as a hook, or else he was just seeking revenge for the scare Sandy had given him.

Sandy had heard him one night at his house next door. He got up, and saw the guy's arms sticking through his kitchen window, feeling all over the counter for something he could take. Sandy snuck up on him, grabbed his arms, and yanked him up against the bars on the window, then he screamed in his face, "God knows what you're doing!"

It scared the thief so badly that he screamed too, only in real fear! Sandy didn't have any way to secure him, so he had to let him go. He wore us and the dog out, and when we went to sleep, he got what he wanted anyway!

October 23, 1987 Tonopah, Nevada

Our thief did return on the night I had left to go home to Nevada for a month. He knew I would be gone, and he knew Flo wouldn't hear him. He broke the bars on the dining room window, and made a hole in the screen, but didn't get in. Wilber, and Sandy's night-watchman woke Flo up – I don't know how – and then they slept the rest of the night on the floor in our house.

A hurricane hit Haiti that night, but by the time it came from the south, over the mountains, it had pretty well broken up, and was more of a tropical storm when it hit Cap-Haitien. When I went to the airport, I didn't even know a hurricane was coming, but the MFI pilot said he was in a hurry to get away before it got there.

I have been here in Tonopah, Nevada a full month now, and I plan to be back in Cap-Haitien on November third. I will be going to see my Kathy and Tony in Maryland for two days on my way back to Haiti.

I went with my mom to California on the sixth of October, and stayed until the twelfth. My mom went on a bus trip to Arizona with the Super Sixties class from Grace Church, and I stayed with my Aunt and slept on her couch.

While I was there, I drove all over looking for supplies for my new clinic. I didn't know how, or where I would get them, but I knew the Lord would do it, if I made myself available – and He did!

Before I left Tonopah, I called Al Mount to let him know I was coming to California, and he told me about a place in Upland called REAP International. They recondition hospital equipment, and then sell it to missionaries cheap. I drove out there, and got a micro- hematocrit centrifuge, a baby scale, and a table top sterilizer, all of which only cost me four hundred and fifty dollars, but it would have been a lot more if I had to buy it new. They also gave me some cases of baby gavage tube feeding sets, a case of four by four wound dressing gauze pads and some syringes and needles, so it was well worth the drive there.

I had several meetings at Grace Church, and one was with an elder, Jim George, who had just come back from Haiti. He and another elder had arrived in Haiti the evening of the Tuesday I had left. I didn't know

240

they were coming, but they went to help Pastor Cebien with his Pastor's Conference. While they were there, he told them about his family problems. I am so glad, because it was honest of him, and now they won't hear it from some other source. Also, they really want to help him, and God willing, Maybe they will be able to help him more in his ministry.

It turned out that Jim George is a pharmacist! While he was there, he got very interested in what the clinic would be, and wants to help by sending medicine! Praise the Lord!

How exciting to trust Him and know He will take care of our needs. What a great, glorious God we serve, He is so faithful! Amen!

November 4, 1987 Back in Haiti

One day back in Haiti, and it's as though I had never been away! I arrived back yesterday, and it was so good to see again those I've come to love here, Flo, Kathy and Alice and many others as well. I was disappointed to not see Pastor Cebien, but was not surprised. I learned that Dr. Benson was here, but that he was leaving that day for Port-au-Prince and then home.

I have so many mixed feelings, so many things to learn, and so many of them about myself. I also learned that Flo, Kathy and Alice, and Pastor Cebien will all be leaving on the tenth, and I will be here alone for at least two weeks. Pastor is going to see his family in Miami, Florida, and to perform a wedding on the nineteenth, but who knows when he will return. I wouldn't mind so much, but we have this persistent thief who is intent on getting into this house, and for the first time since I've been here, I feel some twinges of fear.

Also, the political situation could flare up at any time and become ugly, and being alone here might not be the best idea. I talked to pastor about it, and he said to wait until he comes back from Port on Sunday, and he would tell me what I should do. When I came home and told Flo how I felt about the situation in the country, she got angry and said she would stay home then, because she wouldn't leave the house empty. I would never want to cause her to miss her trip, so I told her I will stay and consider it the Lord's will for me.

I went to clinic this morning in Belle Hotesse, and remembered that one of the reasons I had been ready to go home for awhile was because of the pain I feel when I see all the suffering here, not just the people, but of every living creature in this land.

As I flew over the island coming in, I thought of how it looked like a great gentle beast, whose life blood was slowly oozing out of it and into the sea; brown and reddish colored mud flowing in swirls far out to sea, discoloring the blue water. This is the result of the wounds given it by the multiplying parasites who live on it. Like all parasites, they will eventually kill their host, and then, they too will die. It's so sad to see such a beautiful place slowly dying, and because of that, it's slowly killing all the creatures living on it.

November 10, 1987

I went to Diana's clinic this morning, and after about an hour, she called me into the treatment room and asked me to listen to a baby's chest, and give her my opinion. The baby girl was about three months old, beautiful, but very sick. She had some respiratory distress, her color was poor, her eyes were staring, and she had no muscle tone. They had been giving her oral rehydration solution for a while. I really felt uncomfortable about her, and said that I thought she looked like she might die any minute.

I went back to consulting in the other room, but Diana called me back. I stood and looked at the baby, and while I was looking at her, she stopped breathing. Her heart rate began to drop, and I began doing heart massage right there with the baby still in the mother's lap. Then I picked her up and rushed – again – to the other room where there was a table to lay her on. As I continued chest compressions, she vomited a large amount of fluid. We had no suction equipment at all, not even a bulb syringe. Brave Diana went ahead and started breathing for her, but we got no response at all. After about fifteen minutes we made the decision to stop.

The baby had died, and we could not get her back. The mom was called in, and it was terrible! She screamed and cried – understandably, but it really scared the other moms. Wilber took the mom and the baby to the hospital and now our only comfort in our failure to save her was, we knew where she was-safe in the arms of Jesus.

She was just one more tiny Haitian who will never be hungry or sick again; one small, beautiful little black face for the loving Father to smile upon. How comforting to know that when we try so hard to keep them here, He knows what is best, and sometimes He says, "No, I want her back today." Now, she will forever be with the One who gave her life, and the One who has the right to ask for its return. But for those of us who tried to keep her here – it was shattering!

November 11, 1987

Today was Flo's remote clinic in a place beyond San Raphael. She was driving, and we had a car full, but we stopped in San Raphael and picked up Pastor Livingston, and one of Flo's village health workers, and on we went.

The road began to get smaller and very bad with big slippery, gooey, muddy areas. We slipped and slid through several before the next one caught us. We had to get out and put the Rocky into four wheel drive, then with about ten people pushing us, we finally got out. This happened twice, but we finally made it to the clinic.

Our clinic didn't last long, as there were only thirty-three people to be seen. Someone told us that if we went home a different way, it wouldn't be so bad. I figured the known was preferable to the unknown, and I was driving this time. I had learned how to keep two wheels on dry ground, and make it through, but Flo decided we should go the unknown way. We got through one big muddy area, and were going along just fine when we went around a tree, the road disappeared beside the river, and we slowly sank into the mud.

It took an hour and a half of strenuous struggle by several men and lots of little boys; all cheered on by at least thirty on-lookers, before we were finally free of the mud. We weren't sure where to go when we got out as there was no visible road anywhere, so since I was driving now, away we went, down into the river. The water was two to three feet deep, but the bottom was rocky sand instead of mud. Finally, I drove up onto a big gravel bar, around a woman washing clothes, crossed another bit of river, made a quick right up a pretty steep bank, and we were finally back on a road. They were right, it was a better road – at least from that point on!

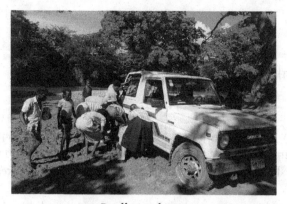

Really stuck!

Then, just to top off the day – I was taking a shower and had just gotten my hair all lathered up, and off went the water! Oh, well, another day in Haiti. And on the way home – I hit a chicken-awful!!

November 22, 1987

One week from today is the BIG day here in Haiti – Election Day! Only God knows what the outcome of that day will be. I hear there is an anti-American feeling in the country, but I'm not really afraid. My life is in the hands of the One I serve. I know that before anything can touch me, it must first pass through His hands of love, but I pray for the sake of this country and it's people, the day will come and go without bloodshed.

Pastor Cebien should return on the twenty-sixth, but I will believe he's back when I see his face. He will probably be in Port on the Sunday of elections, so I don't know when I'll see him again.

I am praying for Diana and her husband John. He is leaving to look for work in the States, as he feels demeaned here. All of his business ventures have failed, and he cannot support his wife and himself. She has chosen to remain here with her four Haitian children. I hope they are not making a big mistake.

Later entry: February 12 1988 I have learned that John cannot stay in the States because he cannot produce either a death certificate or a divorce paper from his first wife. He may still be married to her. They have put a hold on both Diana and John, and they are not allowed to leave the country from either airport until they pay their bills. It's really sad to see a good ministry and a person destroyed so easily.

November 26, 1987   Thanksgiving Day

I was invited to two different places for dinner, but I finally decided I didn't want to go anywhere, as I was feeling guilty about the abundance of food we missionaries have when the Haitians have nothing. I had just happily finished my beans and onion bread, when Don Davis came to get me. He said they were waiting dinner for me, and that no one could eat until I got there. I really didn't want to go, but after that message – what could I do? I went, but felt badly. All I could think of was – here we are, a bunch of Americans stuffing our faces, while outside, those we came to 'serve' were starving. Then, after dinner, we had to watch a movie on Lois' new video player. I guess I am being too hard on these folks, they work very hard for these people, and they deserve a day off now and then.

Diana had also invited me, and I almost died laughing when Sandy told me about her turkey. They bought it live, and when the Haitian girl prepared it to cook, she cut it up like you would a chicken, as that's the way they do it here. They don't have a pan or an oven big enough to cook a whole turkey.

When Diana saw it, she got very upset, so Sandy went over and sewed it back together with RED embroidery thread! What a riot!

A tarantula is back on the porch, heading for the dog, who is sleeping there, and beyond, for our open door. I shut the door, but he stayed out there for a long time. Maybe he's catching bugs under the light. He was as big as my hand. They walk so slow and deliberate– picking up one leg at a time, but I've seen them move very fast as well and someone told me these big ones can jump five feet!

November 29, 1987   Election Day

What a very sad day for Haiti this has been! After waiting so long to be able to vote, the day finally came, and they were told – after much bloodshed – that the elections were canceled 'until further notice,' whatever that means. Radio Soleil's station in Port-au-Prince was blown up with a hand grenade, and some who had started to vote were machine gunned. The ballots and voting booths were destroyed.

It looks as though the ones who are in power intend to stay there at any cost. Port-au Prince was a battlefield, but, amazingly, Cap-Haitien was as peaceful as though nothing out of the ordinary was going on. It's so strange that two cities in the same small country could be so different.

I wonder what will happen now? But then, I wonder that every morning when I wake up in this place.

December 11, 1987

Last night, I was just about asleep, when the dog's barking woke me. I heard the night watchman talking to someone, so I got up to see. It was our neighbor in the front house saying that I had a long distance phone call.

I went with him, and to my total surprise, it was my son, Tom. Now Tom had been raised as a Catholic by his step-mother, spending all of his school years in Catholic schools. We talked for awhile, and then he told me that he had decided what he would do with the rest of his life. I asked him, "What?"

His answer was, "I've decided to become a Jesuit priest."

I felt like I'd had a bucket of ice water dumped on me. I didn't know what to say. I wasn't prepared for that. I felt as though I had really failed him, and hadn't prayed enough for him. All I could think of to say was, "That's interesting."

He laughed and said, "That's just what Grandma said." I shouldn't wonder!

January 8, 1988   First Entry of the New Year.

Christmas has come and gone, and the days are all pretty much the same. We've had so much rain, we've had to cancel a lot of clinics. I got my prayer letter written, and sent off to everyone yesterday.

Kathy and Alice were to arrive back here in Haiti on the fifth, but their pastor wanted them to wait until after the elections are over here. They are now scheduled for the seventeenth.

We're hearing rumors of expected fighting and blood shed to come, but they're saying that it won't come to Cap.

I can't drive the Rocky into town, because it doesn't have a windshield sticker – someone took it, and then a week ago, someone stole the papers for the car out of the glove compartment, so without them, I can't even buy a sticker.

The clinic at Morne Rouge is coming along, but as usual, there is always a problem of money. I have boxes stacked up in two corners of my room with supplies for it.

Winston, from South Africa, was here (I met him last year) and he's taken my list of 'needs and wants' home to his church. Perhaps the Lord will use some of them to help us.

Joyce has been going on the remote clinics very faithfully with me. Today, we went to La Brié, and our first patient, a six month old baby girl died before we had a chance to help her. She'd been sick for eight days, was unresponsive to the penicillin shot I gave her, and she just quit breathing, and went into the arms of Jesus. It was heart rending.

The poor parents had walked for two hours to get there, and now they would have to carry her little body all the way back up into the mountains where they lived. They were told by those around, not to cry as they went, because if they did, people would want to see, and it would take them much longer to get home.

Later, as we were working, we began to hear loud wailing, crying and lamenting. It was a funeral coming down out of the mountains. It was for Pastor Dorléon's aunt, so we were without his, or his brother's, help today.

That was the second funeral of the day. While we were walking to the clinic, and were just about there, another funeral went by with the coffin, the wailers, and all.

The thing about Haitian funerals is this, the louder you wail, tear your hair and cry, the more you are showing how much you cared for that person, so it's important to make a lot of noise, but it is rather unnerving to hear it. It sounds like the whole crowd is dying!

As we were nearing the finish of the clinic, a lady came running, carrying a little boy of about four or five years old. He had a deep gash on the top of his head from a machete. His father had been cutting down trees, and the little boy just ran right into the danger, as little kids will, and his father had accidentally hit him with the machete. It was bleeding profusely, so we put a pressure dressing on it, and Joyce took him to the mission doctor to have it stitched up. The doctor put six stitches in it, and Joyce brought him back. He was groggy from a sedative the doctor had given him, but was hopefully going to be okay.

It was about 1:30 when we got home; it was quite a day! I was rather expecting a couple of missionaries today to bring the beautiful oak desk I bought from some friends to the house for me. It's perfect for my room, and it will be nice to get this wide table out of here, which will give me more room. Maybe they'll bring it tomorrow.

January 10, 1988

My daddy would have been 81 years old today, but he's been in Heaven for six years now, waiting for the rest of us to join him.

I hear the drums tonight; haven't heard them for awhile. We're also hearing rumors about trouble this next week, because of the elections on Sunday, but we hear rumors all the time, and so far, nothing has happened here, thank the Lord! I'm going to go with Sandy tomorrow, and get some food stocked up just in case we can't get to the store next week. It seems to be shaping up to be a battle between the military and the people.

January 24, 1988

Well, the elections have come and gone, and there was no trouble. They say there is a new President, but they have yet to say what his name is.

Flo is home, and things are getting back to normal.

Sandy is housing a team of thirteen adults, including Darlynn's mom and dad. The others are members of the congregation from her dad's church; he's a pastor, in up-state New York. They've come to work on her clinic. Flo and I were invited to come over and share their evening devotions; I've gone over a couple of times, and it was enjoyable.

Today, I went with the group to the Citadel, the huge stone fortress way up on the top of a mountain. We drove part way up the mountain, and then most of them rode horses the rest of the way up. I felt too sorry for the poor little skinny horses, so I walked, along with three others. I just barely made it. I had one guide pushing from behind, and another pulling from the front. It was really very funny! I think it was even worse than the hike with Pastor Cebien to the other Belle Aire! When we got to the top, the view was magnificent! One could see for miles and miles.

The Citadel is a big stone fortress, with what looks like the prow of a ship overlooking the whole countryside below. It was built by one of the first 'kings' of Haiti, during the Revolution there, which freed them from the French. The view from the top was spectacular, and the trip down was much easier, but I believe this is another one of those – once is enough events.

January 29, 1988

I feel that I am having a serious problem with my wrong responses to some of the things happening here. Richard, 'the begger' brought in tons of stuff for Flo – food and medicines especially. The last time he brought stuff, Flo was gone, and he said that some of the medicines were for me. I sorted it all out, put it all away for Flo, and I took some of the medicines for my clinic. Tonight, he came for dinner, and Flo had also invited another missionary, who had never met Richard before. She asked him for some of the stuff he brought, and he had two boxes for her. He brought nothing for me, though I have told him several times, when he has asked, that I need medicines for my clinic. I have been helping Flo for two days, sorting clothes she brought back with her to give away, and now there's all of this stuff!

I guess I'm just feeling sorry for myself, having a 'pity party', and I know that is NOT pleasing to the Lord. I have to remember that these are all Flo's projects, yet she's been willing to include me in them. When I asked her if maybe I could have some of the pediatric medicines – not all of them, just to share a few with me, her comment was, "Oh, I don't take care of any kids, right?!" I gave her a hundred dollars the other day, because she was short; I try to help her all I can, and this is what I get – sarcasm!

"Lord, please keep me sweet and loving as you were, even when you were so unappreciated. Help me to remember that I am serving You, and that You have said that You will supply ALL my needs – in ways, and through means that I don't even know. Amen!"

February 1, 1988

Praise the Lord, my little 'pity party' is over. We had three days and nights of rain with no let up. These little mud huts don't do very well in water, and the people can't get out to buy, or sell. Because of this, they were running out of food, and were coming to our door for anything we could spare. Because the Lord knew, and His timing is perfect, we were able to give them all some food. It wasn't what they were used to, but it was easy to fix, and it was food. We had two large Pampers boxes full of dry chicken and rice soup, two cases of soda crackers, and a fifty pound bag of oatmeal; all nourishing food that the whole family could eat. The Lord is so good, and it was such a blessing to see them smile when they got what they needed.

February 9, 1988

Today's mail has made my heart rejoice, and overflow in gratitude and praise to our Almighty God. He is the Almighty One, and yet He has bent down, all the way down to me, here in Haiti. He has literally showered me with answers to prayer. In today's mail I received:

1. From Laerdal Medical, I received a letter from the President of the company saying that they were sending me eight brand new ambu bags (for resuscitation breathing) two of each size, adult, child, and infant; all with several sizes of masks for each bag. In their letter they said that they had read that I had no suction equipment, so they sent a portable suction machine, with suction tubing of every size. A respiratory therapist at the hospital where I had worked, had read my prayer letter, and had sent it to this company, and this was their response! Praise the Lord!

2. A friend of my mother told me that she would like to send me the money I need to finish the clinic, or for a car for me here. Her mother had died, and she had inherited a large amount of money, and she wanted to give some for the Lord's work. Praise the Lord!

3. A friend of mine at Grace Church said in the letter he wrote to me, that John had read part of my prayer letter in church on a Sunday evening. Amazing!

4. I received three cases of liquid Tylenol for children, and one of erythromycin, from someone in Alabama, thanks to the Lord using Winston. The man is a used car dealer, and his daughter is a doctor. Praise the Lord!

These things confirm in my heart that God is in this endeavor, and that it IS His will. I just pray that this clinic will be to His glory, and that His love and compassion will be evident in those who labor there for Him. This is our reason and our motive behind this clinic.

"Flow through us in Your love, and in Your healing power to these poor children of Haiti! And greatly bless those who have given to this effort, for Your glory!"

February 12, 1988

We had a good clinic today at La Brié, even though we got a late start. Since Haiti has a new President, the schools have opened again, and the place we were using for a clinic is now a school. We had to move a little farther up the hill, where we consulted in a Haitian house, and our pharmacy was outside on a table under some trees.

Joyce had the back room where she did treatments. She's really good at it. Today, she lanced a big boil on a little girl, redressed a badly cut finger, dressed a burn, and tried to treat a little boy with kwashiorkor which is a lack of protein. He was so apathetic that he refused to eat or drink anything, and seemed to be in a lot of pain. When his mother tried to force him to drink, he fought and yelled, "Amway, Bon Dieu!" ("Help me, God!") He was no more than four or five years old, which made me wonder, where he had heard that expression.

At one point, Joyce called me and said there was a tarantula on the wall of her 'executive suite', but it was not a tarantula, only a big spider. A little later, a mouse skittered around the corner and into a hole, and Joyce yelled, "It's a baby rat!"

There was a skinny little puppy who wandered through looking for anything someone might have dropped. He gobbled up a bite of a cookie that we had given to a child, and hungrily looked for more.

I don't know how many people we saw, Maybe a hundred plus, but we weren't finished by 1pm. We've decided to try to go there two times a week instead of one. I drove there and back, and crossing the rivers is always a thrill; the banks are so muddy and slippery, and in one place, the bank has not much slope to it, but rather just drops off.

Pastor Cebien asked me if I was ready to start in my new clinic next week! I asked him if he had cabinets built yet, and he said no. He said he'd bring someone from Port to do it. Maybe by the end of March, and that will make it one year that I've been waiting!

February 17, 1988

Many things are happening. We had a good clinic today at Belle Hotesse, and ended with Joyce taking a mother with five week old twins, a two year old boy with kwashiorkor and a little girl about six or seven (the mother doesn't know how old her children are) home with her. They were at the clinic a week ago, and we had started treating the little two year old boy for kwashiorkor, but today he was worse. He had more edema in his legs and feet than previously, and today his penis and scrotum were all swollen. Joyce took him to Dr. Hall, and he said the boy should be hospitalized, so Joyce took the mom and all her kids to her house, where she has a place outside for them to stay.

The little girl was not sick, so Joyce dropped her off at Morne Rouge and left her as Kathy and Alice said they would look after her. They gave her a couple of dresses, some panties, and some shoes and socks. She was thrilled, and right after that, it was lunchtime for the orphans, and she got a big plateful of food. The mother had said that the only food she had to give them was what her neighbors gave her, and they were as poor as she was. Sometimes, they had no food at all, and when they did get some, she must have eaten it all, as the kids were all protein deficient and had the typical red hair of kwashiorkor.

The plight of people here is so sad, and it's getting worse all the time. Food prices keep going up, and at times, even if you had some money to buy food, there is none available to buy, and it's the children and the old who really suffer.

I called Jim and Pam today, and I've decided to go home in March instead of May. This will be better in terms of opening the clinic, and I will surprise my mother on her eightieth birthday. I won't tell her I'm coming, and then I'll just appear on her doorstep and say, "I have a singing telegram for you from Haiti!" Then I'll sing Happy Birthday for her.

Then, when I come back in April, I'll open the clinic, and then I won't leave again until December. I had a good talk with Pastor Cebien, and he agrees.

I went to see Kathy and Alice the other day, and they were sitting in their living room with one of the smaller orphan girls. No one looked very happy, and I thought perhaps there was a discipline problem, but that was not the case. The child was being taken away from the orphanage by her grandfather, because her father wanted her.

She had been brought to them by her mother when she was a three year old in diapers, because her mother knew that she was dying, and wanted the child cared for. The girl has been in the orphanage now for two years, and can't remember any other home. Her grandfather has been looking in all the orphanages for her, and finally found her here, so Kathy and Alice have to let her go, which is very sad. The child has just recently begun to smile, and now she has to go live in Port-au- Prince with her father and two older sisters. The main concern is that she will come to know the Lord, so we'll pray that she will have that opportunity as she grows.

Later note, February 25

After a week, Joyce took the mother she was keeping and her children back home. The two year old boy was much improved, though Joyce said she had discovered that the main problem was an immature selfish mother, who took all the food for herself, and used the little girl as a servant.

There is no answer to the problem, but Christ. Only He can change people's hearts.

February 26, 1988

The clinic is looking good, and Pastor Ceblen seems to be very proud of it. Scott is going to build the cabinets for me, so I can leave for a month and not worry about that.

Flo's second level class has started, but last night it rained all night, so we couldn't have the clinic at La Brié today. Her hearing aid has gone bad, so she is without any as her other one is already in the States for repair. I've had to yell at her all day, and then I forget, and find myself yelling at Ma'Louie, too.

I read a book titled, 'Revolution in World Missions' by K. Yohannan. He is Indian, and his fresh, objective look at missions has really set me to thinking. What he says about ours being a 'social' gospel is so true. And so true, too, is that isn't what saves people. We seem to be going at it backwards. We are using the social work to gather people to evangelize, when we should be evangelizing, and then charging the local church with the social end of it. This would work in the U.S., but in a country like Haiti, the local church itself is in such dire need, and has no resources to do their own social work.

I think I may stay for a couple of years, train someone to take my place, and leave. I'll go home, work, and send money to support Haitian pastors. I hate living so far above what these poor people can have, and yet, they would think I was really crazy if I went to live in a mud hut like they live in. It is really a complex situation

February 27, 1988

I think the 'honeymoon' for Haiti and me is about over. Things that were exciting and stimulating are becoming routine and hum-drum, but that's okay; I really felt it tonight when the lights went off again, just as we were finishing dinner. Flo said, "It's right behind you on the ledge," meaning the matches, but my first thought was – a rat! The lights have been going off every evening about 5:30 or 6pm, and staying off until about 8:30 or 9pm.

Pastor Cebien has the yellow "Lemonzine" back again finally, without the top rack on the roof, which I know he will miss, but Maybe he won't be able to load it down so much. The tires are bald. I just pray that the Lord will protect him in it!

March 3, 1988

I am sitting here writing this by kerosene lamp, as once again, the electricity is off. The scurrying of rats overhead sounds like a race with about a hundred contestants. It almost sounds like they have a race track up there, as they go around and around. Nikki's head just swivels, and her eyes get so big; she can almost taste them!

Today has been very tiring and I'm sorry to say, not exactly all in His service. Sandy's dog, and the neighbor's big brown dog are both in love with the same little girl dog, and this has led to innumerable vicious, bloody fights between the two dogs. I finally couldn't stand it anymore, so I brought Sandy's dog in the house. Even though he cried and cried to go out, I kept him in, and by the end of the day, I felt like I had been baby-sitting a naughty two year old all day long. I was exhausted!

Sometime this morning, one of Flo's students who works at Diana's clinic, brought a woman here to the house, with a very tiny, seven month preemie that had been born yesterday. She couldn't have weighed over two pounds, and she was ice cold to touch, so I know her blood sugar was probably non-existent, plus she had had nothing by mouth since she had been born, more than 24 hours ago. I don't know what her temperature was, but she needed to be warmed up, so I put a towel in the oven, and when it was warm, I wrapped the baby in it, and put another towel in the oven, and for two hours, I rotated them every five or ten minutes. I finally got her warmed up and took her temperature and it was a good 99.2! Praise the Lord!

Next I got a feeding tube, mixed up some half strength formula and started teaching the Aunt who had brought her, how to feed her. The baby seemed to have a lot of mucus, so I showed the Aunt how to use a bulb syringe. The Aunt seemed to learn very quickly, and showed me she could do it. She told me the mother of the baby had had three babies, and they have all died except this one, and she will live only by God's grace and mercy, but then don't we all? She had a good color, though slightly pale, and a tiny expiratory grunt, but she had no heart murmur. If they can keep her warm, and she can tolerate the formula, and doesn't get an infection – she may live!

March 5, 1988

Damien came by to tell me that the tiny baby had died. I'm not at all surprised – she was just too tiny to make it. Damien was all teary eyed; it's nice to see a seventeen year old with such a tender heart

I think the dog fights are over – Praise the Lord! But Flo and I seem to be back in the place where everything I do seems to irritate her. My giving annoys her, she claims I'm making welfare people out of them. She can't stand Ronnie, or Damien, or Wilson – all of whom come around frequently just to talk. Then, there are the dogs - !

It really concerns me. I try to do as much as I can to help her, but sometimes it seems all she focuses on are the things that annoy her. Reminds me of my mother; I must be a very annoying person.

One of the men that stayed at Sandy's with the team from New York, Skip Bramhall, phoned me yesterday – it was a surprise, and he said he wants to meet me in California, and go to Grace Church with me. That will be nice, I guess.

Our hot water heater seems to have died, so I took a bath tonight like I used to do in Port-au-Prince – I heated the water in a pan, and took it in the bathroom, got in the shower, and took my bath in the pan. Great! I've also learned to brush my teeth in just a glass of water.

We had a great clinic yesterday – must have seen a hundred and thirty to a hundred and fifty people, some of whom were really sick with malaria.

March 18, 1988 Tonopah, Nevada

I've been in Tonopah for nine days now. I arrived the night before my mom's birthday, and surprised her by appearing on her doorstep at 8am on her birthday! I went to Bible study with her, and we had dinner at Jeff and Donna's that evening. We came home to have desert, and found at least fifty people here for a surprise party! Even I was surprised!

My mother's friend, Ginny, her husband, and their two little kids came to stay over the weekend. Ginny told me she is giving me three thousand dollars! Praise the Lord! The week has been a good one of visiting and resting. I've had three letters, and three phone calls from Skip. I can't believe this guy! I really don't know what to think about him. All I know about him now, is that he's very persistent!

I tried to change my ticket to stay longer, but found out I can't, so I'll have to go back to Haiti on the 31st as planned.

April 4, 1988   Haiti

I've been back in Haiti since the first of April. I spent a very hectic and wonderful week in California, though it ended with the theft of my little 1980 Honda Accord.

I had let my mom take it to go shopping while I was at Grace Church all day. When she got finished with her shopping, she went to her sister's house, took her packages out of the trunk, and closed the lid down, only she forgot to take the keys out of the lock. Someone came along, saw the keys dangling there, and away went my car. Praise the Lord, it's His car, and He knows all about it. I left the next morning on the plane, so I still don't know if it's been recovered or not.

My time with Skip was pleasant, and bitter sweet. He is a dear, sweet, sensitive, kind, loving, considerate, and generous man, who truly loves the Lord. But, for me, I know there is no other way than the way I am going right now. I have to say, though, that it is a lovely warm feeling to know that there is someone who cares about what happens to you, and who wants to love you with Christian love, which is self-sacrificing service.

Here are the goals set for me by the elders at our meeting on March 31:

1. I have until August to be in and operating the clinic. If it hasn't happened by then, I must start thinking about going elsewhere, some other area of service, either in Haiti, or another country.
2. I must go to Port-au-Prince once a month to see Al Warren, and be more accountable to him. There is also a missions meeting in Port once a month, that I should go to, to acquaint myself with other aspects of medical work here in Haiti.
3. I must get into more aggressive language study, such as getting a tutor.

April 5, 1988

It's mail day, and I received a letter, a picture, and a check from my son, Tom, and his novitiate brothers. They are on their way to becoming Jesuit Priests, but I feel the Lord will draw my son out of the web he is in, and set his feet on the one and only Way.

My heart is sore tonight, because Ronnie and Wilson both came by to see me, and Flo was very unkind, and rude to them both. She jumped up from her chair when they came in the door, and loudly said, "Maybe I should look for another place to live, as this is a marked house where all the beggars and 'riff-raff' come."

I asked her if she would like me to move, but she said, "No, it is the house, and they'd still come." Every day, I get remarks about the dogs, and now, this. Ronnie needs the Lord, and that's why I'm here, or at least I thought that was the reason, because people need the Lord. Wilson is my brother in Christ, and neither of them have sinned any more than I have, or Flo either for that matter. Praise God, that He doesn't slam the door in your face when you make a mistake. It's been like this since I came back on Friday. *"Keep me sweet, Lord!"*

April 7, 1988

Flo is really upset with me. Today on the way home from the airport, she told me I couldn't even live like a missionary, because I wanted 'home baked bread'. I don't really know what that has to do with anything, or if it's worse than having to have a Lazy-Boy recliner shipped all the way to Haiti, but evidently, she feels it's not being sacrificial or something, even though Ma'Louie has been baking bread for Flo since before I ever came here.

When Ronnie came, she got up out of her Lazy-Boy with a crash again, stomped off to her room, and slammed her door! Pretty obvious to both Ronnie and I how she felt. Poor Ronnie was very hurt.

We have a night watchman, and tonight I warmed up a tiny bit of weenies and beans that were left over, because the half sandwich I had fixed for him looked like so little, and she came out and accused me of playing 'one-upmanship'. I really don't know what to think, or do. Thank the Lord that He knows the motives for the things I do, and 'one-upmanship' is not my motive for doing anything. How petty and unworthy of Him it would be to have such a motive. I do confess that I'm having a difficult time wanting to help her with her clinics. My love is not very evident right now, in that I don't feel like self-sacrificing service for her, which is where I am wrong.

I bought a car today from a lady from Porto Rico. She has the dairy here, where we buy wonderful fresh pasteurized milk. Any way, she sold me this little yellow Datsun for three thousand dollars. I gave her three hundred dollars down, and I'll pay her a hundred dollars a month. Praise the Lord! I'll call it the 'Ti-Limo'. (Little Limo)

April 11, 1988

Every day has become a heavy hearted one, with little jabs and pokes given verbally to me all day long. I went and had a good talk with Kathy and Alice about it, but it looks like the only way I'll ever have peace with Flo, is to tell Ronnie and Wilson to stay away, and – kill the dogs! I really don't know what to do. I don't know what she wants from me, or what she wants me to do. I'd do it if I knew.

I got my car tonight about 9:30. The lady I bought it from drove it over, and asked me to drive her home again. So- I got in, and drove her back to her house, and we ran out of gas in her driveway! She put five gallons in for me, and I came home. She also said the spare was flat. Praise the Lord that I didn't run out of gas after I was on my way home again, as I'd have been stranded somewhere between her house and home, which would have been a pretty long walk.

April 12, 1988

I washed three days worth of dirty clothes by hand today, as our washer is leaking, then I went to the airport for our mail at 10:30, but the plane didn't come until 12:45. It was really hot in the airport, but I had a chance to talk with a man from another mission down the road about Ronnie and Wilson. From what he says, and all the other missionaries say, I guess I'll have to tell Wilson to stay away. He said, however, for Ronnie, he had a job for him, translating written English into Creole. Praise the Lord!

When the plane came in, I found that the dog food I ordered didn't come, and a box with books and tapes seems to be lost; I didn't hear from any of my family, and when I got home, my white dresses I had washed were on the ground. Wilson came by, and I had to tell him not to come anymore. I felt like a traitor!

I looked for Ronnie, but couldn't find him, so when Damien came by, I sent him to look for Ronnie and give him the note I had written telling him to come and see me. He came in the evening, and I took him to meet the missionary who would give him a job.

My car has a very bad shimmy when it gets up to a certain speed. I hope I didn't make a mistake in buying it, and I hope it will last until I get it paid for.

The electricity has been off since 7pm, and it's now 9:15, and it's really hot, and NO fan. I'm melting! I feel like the Lord is heating up the furnace ten times hotter, and I am suddenly finding myself trying to take joyfully the 'spoiling' of my goods. It seems like since the night my car was stolen, everything has gone wrong.

I had taped some really beautiful music, and I really loved it, because it made me happy to listen to it. I tried to play it today, and found that I must have erased it taping some other music. I was really unhappy with myself.

We went to Pastor Maizamo's clinic this morning, but neither Joyce nor Claud showed up to help us, so we were short.

We saw the usual one hundred plus people, but we had a girl of about ten with leprosy on her face. Flo went and got the medicine for it at Limbé

Hospital. It takes one forth of a pill of Dapsone two times a week for her. Sure doesn't seem like much for such a terrible disease.

I drove my car some more today, and it shimmies when I go over 35 mph. I knew I should have driven it before I bought it, but I trusted the owner. I don't know why I'm so trusting; I guess Maybe naive would be a better word!

I feel like I am losing heart and becoming discouraged. This does not glorify Him at all, nor does it please me.

April 19, 1988

Diana asked me to take her clinic for this Tuesday and Thursday, as she and Darlynn will be in the States. At 7:30 this morning, a man was at the door telling me there were 'ampil moun' at the clinic. (many people) I drove over, and indeed there were. I made my first mistake about two minutes after I arrived.

I said that the clinic was closed, and that I would only see kids with high fevers. It was instant angry panic! They mobbed me, and I could hardly move. They were trying to grab the numbers out of my hand, and I was in big trouble!

I finally gave out twelve numbers, and retreated into the building. There was no way I could leave, so I ended up seeing them all! I was there for seven hours of non-stop crying, sneezing, coughing kids. When it was over, I felt like I had been mugged, and then run over by a truck.

April 20, 1988

Today was clinic at Belle Hotesse, and we had so many people, we ran out of medicines, which meant many unhappy people. When I finally got into the shower this evening, and got my hair wet, the electricity went off! There I was in the dark with my head dripping wet. I managed to get it done by turning the water off between soapings, but before I could get it dry, someone was banging on the front door.

Flo finally answered it, and it was the neighbor in the front saying that I had a telephone call. Oh boy, I didn't even have my clothes on yet. I threw something on, and went running down the drive in the dark.

It was an elder from Grace Church, and while we were talking, someone in the house decided to light the gas stove in the kitchen. There was an explosion that broke glassware, and shook the house. The lady of the house jumped up, yelling, "What happened?" and went running to see. I found out when I hung up, about the stove. No one was hurt - just another night in Haiti!

April 21, 1988

I went back to Diana's clinic for another round. Today, they were much better behaved, and I didn't see but about half of the number I saw the last time. One of the babies was a Down syndrome with a myelomenengecele, which is a failure of the spinal canal to close. Nothing can be done in this country for this baby, and though I gave the mom antibiotics to give her, I'm afraid she will die from an infection before she's a year old.

April 27, 1988

Another week is gone, and I think I've gotten four letters from Skip. No clinic this morning as Joyce had to go to Port-au-Prince to get the braces on her girl's teeth tightened, and Flo left at noon for Thomasique in the mountains. So – I'm here alone, and I have to say it's lovely. I had a good Creole lesson with Lange, my tutor, this afternoon.

This morning, two pretty little green hummingbirds flew into the house, and Nikki, Flo's cat, was beside herself with excitement! I put her in a bedroom and shut the door which really upset her.

I think one was a mama bird, and the other her baby. They were an apple green, and the smaller one had a short tail, and couldn't fly very far. I got the bigger bird out right away, but the small one wasn't quick or smart enough. It finally flew into a door, slid down to the floor where I was able to pick him up in my hand. I carried him out to the hummingbird feeder on the porch, set him on a perch, and curled his tiny feet around it, and left him sitting there in a daze. He finally took off and flew away, but I could hear them calling to each other for quite a while afterwards. He felt so soft and so tiny in my hand, and he was so frightened. How wonderful it will be in the Millenium, when we will be able to touch and hold those sweet little creatures that are now so afraid of us. I can hardly wait!

Nikki was really miffed because we put her in the bedroom, and shut the door so she couldn't get them. We really spoiled all her fun! She looked and looked for those birds – yet she sleeps at night while a rat sits and eats our bananas!

I'll be helping Darlynn on Tuesdays and Thursdays until she leaves. It will be interesting to see how the Lord will work all this out.

May 2, 1988

We went to LaBrié again today from 10am-2:30pm, and it was so hot, I thought I was going to melt into a puddle! Sitting in that mud house, with people blocking the door, was miserable. The sweat just ran down my back, my sides, and my face. Then, when I started feeling sorry for myself, I remembered that those I came to help were sitting there, much hotter than I was. They had fevers, and felt sick besides. Once in awhile a tiny breeze would squeeze by the crowd, and, oh my, did it feel good for a second or two. I would say, "Oh, thank You Lord!" It was wonderful.

I forgot to take some food for the puppy who lives there, so I was feeding him some little cheese crackers, when he threw up on the floor. The owner came and cleaned it up by throwing a shovel full of dirt over it, and then scooped it all up. One advantage of a dirt floor.

When we got home, as I was taking a shower, (Praise the Lord for the shower) I was thinking about Darlynn's clinic. I could do it two days a week, and Pastor Cebien's, two days a week, and go with Flo on her remote clinic the other day. Darlynn said that the mission board of her church pays the rent on the building, and they pay the help as well. There are a lot of things to think about, talk about, and pray about. Grace Church would have to make the final decision for me, and Pastor Cebien doesn't even know about it as he's still not back yet.

May 8, 1988

Friday, we had our clinic on a huge slab of cement that is used to dry rice and cocoa beans. The weather is so humid and oppressive, that the mud hut with the pharmacy under the tree, was just not working. Pastor Dorléon found another place close by, but because it had rained the night before, the embankment was too slippery to climb. His next find was this big slab of cement, which is great!

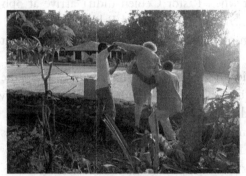

Ronnie and Pastor Dorleon helping Flo over a little wall and onto the cement slab.

We waited while they went around and found tables and chairs, and then we tried to decide where to put them. I told Flo it reminded me of when I was small, playing house – 'the bedroom will be over there, and these will be our chairs over here.' We had sheets hanging to separate the rooms, and we saw about seventy people. Our pharmacy was under a big tree.

On our way home, in the middle of one of the rivers we cross, was a tap-tap stuck in the mud, right in the middle of the river. There was the inevitable one- hundred folks giving advice, and at least fifty, trying to do what the hundred advised. I knew I'd never make it through the mud if I had to slow down to keep from hitting someone, so I started blowing the horn, and inching forward until they all got out of the way, and then I stepped on the gas, and across we went. I'm sure some of them got a muddy water shower, but the banks are steep, and the mud is deep, and I didn't want to get stuck, and have to deal with the hundred!

We learned on Friday, that Pastor Cebien's cousin, Pastor Felix, had been killed – murdered! Then later, we learned that he had been on a tap-tap, on his way to the airport to meet Pastor Cebien, who was coming in from Florida. A gray taxi had pulled the tap-tap over, and told the driver they wanted one of his passengers, and called him by name. Witnesses said that Pastor Felix got out, and went willingly with the five men, as though he knew them. He was never seen alive again.

They began to look for him, and finally, his body was found in a field near the airport. He had been brutally hacked up with a machete. They think that the men were possibly after Pastor Cebien, and were using Felix as a decoy, but when Pastor Cebien didn't arrive at 3pm when he was supposed to, they might have killed Felix, because, now he knew what they were planning, and they were angry at being frustrated in their evil plans.

Pastor Cebien arrived at 10pm that night, as the plane he was on had to return to Miami because of a problem. The Lord knew, even though Pastor Cebien didn't.

He has been threatened before, but the Lord continues to preserve his life. I just wish I knew WHY someone wants to kill him.

Poor Pastor Felix – he was always so nice to me. He always tried to help me with my Creole, and I really liked him a lot. He leaves a wife and seven kids, from fifteen years to five months old. In January, their house burned down, along with a whole block of houses in the dismal area of Port-au-Prince where they lived. Since then, they've been living in one nine by nine room; nine people in a nine by nine room. And we have the audacity to complain about anything!

We're going to Port tomorrow for the funeral. I still haven't seen Pastor Cebien since he's returned. He and Felix were raised together, and were like brothers, so I know this has really hurt him.

We now have a tarantula that lives in the medicine room. Every night he comes out and sits and waits for some dinner to come by. I'm afraid he's going to starve to death. (May 18; He did!)

May 20, 1988

Dr. Benson showed up tonight, and I was going to hide in my room. Flo came and said that he wanted me to come out, and join them. I came out and joined them, thinking to go back in a few minutes.

He gave a discourse on Medical Ambassadors, which he founded; then a Bible study on 'Our thought life'; we had prayer all around, and then he was going to leave.

Before he left, he took me aside, and said he wanted to speak to me. I had no idea what to expect, as he has been pretty negative in his attitude toward me. He had told me that I was not welcome to work with any Medical Ambassadors missionaries, (which Flo is) and, I was not allowed to drive the Rocky, which I did anyway, because Flo's arthritis in her hands makes it painful for her to drive, especially on the rough roads. He also tried to get Flo to make me move out of the house.

We walked into the dining room, and he said that his thoughts about me had not always been kind in the past. He apologized, and asked me to forgive him! I told him that he had been forgiven long ago, but that I appreciated his apology. I also told him that I thought that he was doing a very good work here in Haiti. I was glad, because he's not really a bad man. Praise the Lord, who frequently gives us some hard lessons to learn!

May 24, 1988

Sandy just came over and told us that our main supplier of medicines in town, Pharmacie Du Centre, burned down last night, along with the dry cleaners next door. I was just going to go and buy a thousand dollars worth of medicines for my new clinic! This is a real disaster for the work here, and is bound to cause us problems. We may have to go all the way to Port now to get our medicines, and that will be awful! The Lord knows, and He is still in control.

Kathy and Alice said that one of Pastor Cebien's friends came from Port, and told him, that if he wanted to stay alive, he'd better not go back to Port. She said that someone who knows both sides, came and told her that Pastor Felix was killed because he was so close to Pastor Cebien, and that after they had killed Felix, they went back to the airport to wait for Pastor Cebien to come in, to kill him, but the Lord had other plans, and caused him to arrive much later than expected; he was seven hours late arriving in Port, and they had given up for that time, and had left the airport before he arrived

I asked Kathy and Alice, why did they want to kill him? Evidently, Pastor is a distant relative of the dictator Jean-Claud Duvalier, and was at the palace occasionally. They said that when the three of them were going to Port every weekend, he would be gone all night every Friday night. The government now is no different than when Duvalier was in power, but now it's General Namphy's people, and I guess Pastor Cebien is not one of them. I don't know all the ins and outs of it, but it's not good, I know that! A matter for much prayer!

10pm – Pastor Cebien is leaving for Port tomorrow, and won't be back until Sunday. I just pray he WILL come back! Alive! The last time he went, they were hunting for him, and it was his wife's brother who said that, 'he could die just like Felix did.'

At one point, Pastor Cebien was in another Pastor's car, and he said he just had a 'feeling' that he should move over. He moved, and just then, the car was rammed into by the grey taxi – right where he had been sitting! The pastor who was driving then took him to the bus depot so he could get a bus back to Cap-Haitien. He started to get on one- driven by a friend of his – and he saw the grey taxi again, described as the one that Felix had gotten into. He got out of the bus, got onto an empty one, and hid down on the floor. After awhile, he decided to write down all that had been happening to him, so he sat in a seat, and opened his briefcase to write, when he saw the grey taxi again, so he got back down and hid again. It was a good thing that he hid again, because they came into the bus, but didn't see him, and left. When the bus driven by his friend was nearly full, he went and got on it. Normally, the buses stop here and there, but the driver said that if anybody wanted to stop, they should get off and get on a different bus because he was not stopping, in order to get Pastor Cebien to Cap safely. Pastor had explained to his friend what was happening, and the driver had said, "I'll get you to Cap!"

This afternoon, a letter from Pastor Cebien's wife came on a tap-tap. I just pray she won't unknowingly lure him to Port, and get him killed.

June 3, 1988

Well, Skip came down to visit me, and he's been here for five days so far. Today, he went with us to La Brié, and I have to say, it was nice to have him there. He was sitting on a cement curb watching us as we were seeing our patients. I had just put my stethoscope on a child, when I heard him say, "Will you marry me?" What could I say? I said, "No."

He is a lovely Christian man, but I do NOT feel free to even think about getting married again. I really wish I could make him understand. I think he does, but he says he won't give up. The Lord can change his heart, and I pray He will.

Pastor Cebien has gone to the States again for two weeks. We'll never get that clinic done, and today, I had a letter from Dr. Bibiana, saying that she will be here July third. While I was at Grace Church the last time, one of the elders asked me if I would be interested in having a doctor come down to work with us. I was thrilled, and said, "Oh, yes!" She is from Argentina, speaks English well, and is a specialist in tropical medicine. She is young and single, and wants to come and work with us. Praise the Lord!

June 24, 1988

Skip left after being here for two weeks. We got better acquainted, and learned a lot about each other, while we spent some time together. One of our favorite recreations in the evening, was sitting on the front porch, and watching the rats come out of the attic in the dusk. They come out, run down the wire to the pump, and down to the ground. I've tried to convince the Haitians that one reason they have so many rats, is because they kill all the snakes and eat the cats that would control the rat population – but they're not convinced! They really HATE snakes.

We went to La Brié again, and it was a long clinic. This afternoon, while Flo was gone, Meg brought some folks from the Fort Lauderdale Lion's Club by our house. They brought us some bread, and some other food for us to give away. They wanted our 'wish list,' and they were going to fill it for us. They also invited me to join them, and some other missionaries at the Mont Jolie Hotel for dinner. I should have gone to Bible study, but I didn't go, instead, I went with Sandy, Meg, and the Lion's Club to Mont Jolie and had a good dinner, and talk with these folks. They're not Christians, but nice, well meaning people.

July 3, 1988

Today is the day our Doctor is supposed to arrive in Port-au-Prince. I haven't heard any more from her, so I asked Al Warren if he would meet her plane, keep her overnight, and put her on MAF for Cap-Haitien in the morning. He said he would do it.

Skip called me Friday night and we talked for 45 minutes. In the course of that conversation, he told me what Grace Church had decided in the monthly Outreach meeting regarding my taking over Darlynn's clinic. They said I could try it for three months, and then the situation will be re-evaluated. I'm afraid that I won't be able to do it alone. I'll have the Haitian helpers, but no other nurse. However, I will have a Doctor if Bibiana gets here, at least for July, and then a nurse for August, so that only leaves September, and the Lord knows what's ahead, and I trust Him totally!

July 4, 1988

We had our Grand Opening celebration for the clinic at Morne Rouge tonight. Pastor Cebien talked, and then he and Kathy and Alice sang a couple of songs, which were so nice. I just love to hear them sing! Then he presented me with the keys to the clinic. (After I gave them to him so he could) Then we had an Open House, and showed everyone the clinic. We had some Coke and some cookies, and then Don Davis set off some fireworks he had. Of course, the electricity went off just as we were going to show everyone the clinic, so we showed them by lantern light. (Probably better that way, anyway.) Pastor prayed for the clinic after he gave me the keys. It was very nice.

I will be at Darlynn's on Tuesday, and then Wednesday morning at 8am, I will start here for our first clinic at Morne Rouge. Finally! Now, I have two clinics for children! He gives more grace, and His strength is made perfect in weakness! Amen!

July 6, 1988

Our first day! I had six patients, and I made five dollars and forty cents. I have four people from the other clinic to work here, and I will pay them each four dollars a day. I will pay Ronnie, who is here to translate for me when I need it, out of my pocket, so he will not be employed by the clinic. He and I stayed until 3pm (everyone else was done by 10am) packing pills for next Wednesday's clinic. Francoise in the pharmacy had a hard time as nothing was already packaged, except the samples we had to give out.

Our biggest problem is, we have NO water. There is a nice new sink with a nice counter, but there is no plumbing, and I don't know if there ever will be. We also have no refrigerator. (I could keep vaccines if I had one) but we probably wouldn't have any electricity to run one anyway.

July 7, 1988

I told everybody at Darlynn's that she would be leaving, and I would be taking her place. I have no idea how they feel about it. Their faces were blank, and no one said anything.

July 9, 1988

We went to the airport for MAF's flight from Port-au-Prince, but still no Doctor. I don't know why, but I'm just praying that she is alright.

Today is Sandy's and Skip's birthdays. I took Sandy the cup I'd gotten for him. He told me that Chien, his dog, had gotten in a fight with a bigger dog, and had gotten hurt again. Poor little dog.

July 10, 1988

We went to Pastor Maizamo's church this morning, and after Sunday school, there was to be a baptismal service.

Everyone started out over a little foot path to the ocean and though Flo and I started out with them, we were soon bringing up the rear. The path was winding, and there was tall grass on both sides. I could see just the tops of heads over the grass, winding along like a snake. There was a fellow playing an accordion, and everyone was singing. It looked like Africa.

When we finally got to the beach – it had to be a mile and a half, maybe two – Pastor Maizamo was standing on the muddy beach, with a long white coat on, preaching.

When he finished his message, the accordion and singing began again, while those, who were to be baptized, got ready. Pastor Maizamo and an older lady began wading out into the water, which was about knee deep for a long way out. They went so far out, that I knew if I took pictures, all I would have would be a lot of scenery, with little black dots for people. I decided I would wade out too. I left my shoes on (they were very old ones) and I started out into the water.

The bottom was muddy, and uneven, and I had to step very slowly and carefully, because I was afraid of falling in and ruining my camera. I got way out, but I was still too far away from the action, so I motioned Pastor Maizamo to come back toward me a little, which he did.

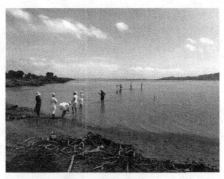

Ocean Baptism

I took some pictures, and then tried to get back to dry land. The mud was sucking the shoes off my feet, which made it hard to keep my balance, but I finally made it back. It was an experience similar to the Citadel – once, was enough. Three little boys had shucked all their clothes off, and gone to play in the water while the baptism was taking place. It was rather funny!

July 11, 1988

I went to the airport again at 9am, but when MAF came in, there was still no Doctor. I will have to call, and see what's become of her.

Later at home, about 5:30 or 6pm, a car drove up, but I didn't recognize anyone getting out - it was raining a bit, and I couldn't see very well. Then, I recognized Marilyn Schaferly, and she had someone with her – our little Doctor!

Instead of taking the plane, she had gotten a ride with some missionaries to Cap-Haitien, and they had taken her to one of the other missions, because she didn't know where I lived. Bless her heart; she's having some experiences already! She's really nice, and such a sweet person. We were SO glad to see her!

August 2, 1988

So much has happened since Dr. Bibiana arrived. I now have two clinics, Babiole, and Morne Rouge, and for awhile, I was really struggling with it all. Bibiana has been a real joy, and a wonderful help. She is always sweet, and willing to help.

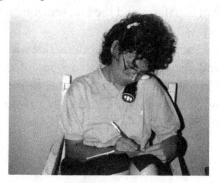

Dr. Bibiana Pinto

My first day at Babiole, someone locked the keys IN the clinic, so we had to pry the bolt off to get in. Then, when the water company – after six months without any – decided to give us water, the faucet in the sink was open, and the stopper was in – so, we had a flood.

Today, we saw a hundred and twenty-five kids, and I had to take time out to take Flo to the airport, and pick up Denise, who was coming to spend some time helping us. She is a very sweet girl, but she has had a terrible introduction to Haiti!

I gave her Flo's room, and she had gone to bed and was asleep, when – a rat fell off of the shutter on the window over her head - right on her face! Poor girl! She came to the door and very quietly said, "There's a rat in my room!" I had told her there were rats in the attic, but I said not to worry, they don't come in the house.

I went in and looked, and sure enough there it was! I couldn't believe it, and the stupid cat just sat and watched it run around. I have hired a night-watchman again, so I called him in, and he chased it all over the room – scared the cat – and the rat finally ran out of the bedroom, and down the hall with the night-watchman right behind it waving his machete. When the rat ran out of the bedroom, Denise and I ran in and shut the screen door so it couldn't run back in there.

The rat ran up inside Flo's Lazy-Boy chair, and the night-watchman finally killed it. (I hope he didn't damage Flo's chair in the process.) Then he brought the rat back down the hall, holding it by its tail to show us – Ugh! All I could say was, "Welcome to Haiti!" I was surprised she didn't leave on the next plane out! I think I would have.

Pastor Cebien invited Dr. Bibiana and me out to dinner, and took us to the Bris de Mer restaurant where we had some wonderful Haitian food. He was a delight as always, when you can get him away from all of his work.

September 4, 1988

It's becoming difficult to keep up with writing in this, so much has happened. Dr. Bibiana and Sandy next door have become quite involved with each other, and now, they are talking marriage! They were so cute at the airport. I've never seen Sandy like this; he seems to be in a trance, with a big smile on his face all the time.

Denise went home on the thirtieth of August, and Skip came again on the twenty-third to stay until the sixteenth of September. He's staying with Scott, another missionary, but he seems to be here at our house all day which doesn't make Flo real happy, I'm afraid.

The electricity situation has gotten so bad; we have as long as thirteen hours at a time without any at all. When this happens, we have no water either, that is, we didn't until now.

Skip built a platform to fit on our peaked roof. Then he put a 30 gallon plastic barrel up there on it, and now when we have electricity, the cistern pump fills the barrel, and we can have a shower even if there's no electricity. It just comes down by gravity! The sun warms the water just enough, and it's wonderful! Especially after a long hot clinic.

I wanted Skip to listen to John's tape on I Corinthians today, so he would know why I didn't feel free to marry again, but the Lord turned the tables on me, and I learned that according to verse 8, those who were divorced and unmarried when they became a Christian, were free to marry again. I have felt for a long time now, that I couldn't have been a Christian until I listened to that tape of John's, and my life was changed. When I think of my life before then, it's just not possible that I was a Christian. Now, I don't know what to do. I thought I had the answer, but now, I don't know. I still don't really want to get married again, and I asked him if he really wanted to be number five! He thinks he does, but I'm still not sure.

September 29, 1988

So much has happened. There has been another coup, in fact there have been two. Manigat was ousted, and Namphy proclaimed himself President. Now, he has been ousted, and an ex-priest named Avril has been elected President, or whatever they choose to call it here. There is a real power struggle going on within the military, and its anybody's guess what will happen next. In the meantime, the poor little people of this terrible place continue their daily struggle – just to survive to the next day. They're not so much concerned with, what is the name of whoever is in power, but rather – will we have any food tonight? Or tomorrow?

On the twenty-first, here in Cap-Haitien, there was a power struggle between the police and the military. We heard guns all day, and into the night. There was a hit list and it was supposedly a list of the competitors of the big man in the drug world. Several were deshoukéd, or killed; some businesses were burned, and several homes were looted and destroyed. It was mob rule. They gave the hit list out, and the mob took over. It's always an unnerving thing to hear gunfire, no matter how far away it is. Actually, I heard it up toward town, and down the other way as well. Shooting continued the next evening as well, but no one seemed to know who was shooting, who they were shooting at, or why they were shooting.

The clinics are keeping me busy, but more and more, I wish I could close Morne Rouge, and just concentrate on Babiole. The Lord knows, and I know that He will do His own perfect will, including changing the minds of the elders concerning Babiole, if that is necessary.

Right now we are without water or electricity in the clinic. I have to make two gallons of Ampicillin syrup a week, plus haul water. We found a dead rat in the drawer of the dossier file cabinet, (what an awful smell!) a tarantula in the latrine, and the road to the clinic is all washed out, with big rocks from the hard rain we've had lately. I can't get over it in my car. I have to park, and then tote everything up to the clinic. I've sent Ronnie to the electric company twice, with no success of finding out what's wrong. Today, I went to see the owner of the building to see if he would help me by going himself, but he wasn't home, and those who were there were rather unfriendly, and no help. Another exercise in futility!

I wish Skip was here, it might be just a fuse or something simple, that I don't know how to fix. We really need the refrigerator. He spoiled me when he was here, and then went and left me alone again.

Yesterday, my car broke down, right in front of the big bus depot, in all that mad traffic. Three men pushed me into the Esso station to get my car in a safe place, and I left the car and walked home. Just this morning, as I backed it out, I thanked the Lord for this good little car, so I guess now, He is testing me. I walked all the way home, several miles, thanking Him, and He was giving me His joy – that unspeakable joy – that this world can never understand.

After dinner, I took the Rocky to Don and Karen's, and they took their SUV and towed my car to their house. Don Davis is a missionary to the missionaries. He's the one who fixes everything for us. Today, he checked it out, and wrote an order for a part for MFI to bring on their next flight. Then he went downtown just to see if maybe he could find the part there, though he was pretty sure he couldn't. He went into a store, wondering how he was going to communicate as he doesn't speak Creole, and 'just by chance' (God planned) the fellow behind the counter spoke perfect English! He also had the part, and said, "It was one twenty-five."

Don thought he meant a hundred and twenty-five, but he meant a dollar and twenty-five cents! So, in less than twenty-four hours, I had my car back again – and I can't believe that there are those who don't believe that our God cares about our everyday needs!

What a great and glorious God! Again, He has proved Himself the ABLE, and FAITHFUL God! How I love and praise Him!

Pastor Cebien is gone to the States again, and I miss him in the clinic in the mornings. He always takes my hand, bows, and says, "Bon jour, Blanc!" and pumps my hand up and down, and I say, "Bon jour, Fre'm!" (Good morning, my Brother!) Sometimes I don't feel that he has kept his reason for wanting me to come and help him – so he could spend more time preaching. It doesn't seem to have materialized, though he is building a new big church at Champin, which he says will also be a trade school where people can come and learn a trade. I don't think I will ever really understand him; he is a very complex man.

October 28, 1988

Tomorrow will be a very, very sad day indeed. Tomorrow, we will bury young Pastor Maizamo. He died Wednesday, October 26, from injuries he received in an accident on his motorbike.

He came to the clinic at Morne Rouge about 9:15, and asked me where Miss Flo was. He said that she had told him that she would come to his clinic at Belle Hotesse that day, and would bring his bag of medicines. He must have misunderstood her, because she went to San Raphael. I gave him my keys, and told him that he could go to the house, and get his meds, so he could go and have his clinic. He took the keys, but he never made it to our house.

Just down the road, in front of another missionary's house, he was hit by a car, and severely injured. His helmet was cracked, and his motorbike totaled.

Amos, the American veterinarian, had come by and picked him up, and had taken him to Dr. Harry at the mission station. Dr. Harry said for him to take him to the hospital, that he was too badly injured for him to be able to do anything for him. So Amos took him then, to the city hospital.

A young man came back to my clinic, and told me what had happened. Ronnie, Pastor Dorléon, and I, immediately went to the hospital to see how he was. We found him in their Emergency Room – semi-conscious, but still responsive. He was lying on a narrow metal gurney with no mattress or sheet on it. He had a Foley catheter in, and that was all they had done.

I asked a man I supposed was the Doctor, what they were going to do for him, and his response was, "Who are you?" I told him I was a nurse and his friend, and I wanted to know what they intended to do for him. He told me that Maizamo probably had internal bleeding, and they would do surgery. He also said that he thought he might have a fractured pelvis, and he had a nasty cut on his forehead, so there was a possibility he might have some head trauma.

At that point, time was passing, and they hadn't done anything. They gave us a list of stuff - IV solutions, IV tubing, tetanus anti-toxin, etc., and we had to go to the pharmacy in town to buy them. The hospital had no supplies at all.

When we brought the supplies back, I looked for my keys in Maizamo's pocket, but they were not there. I finally found them – I was locked out of my house – a man had them, along with Maizamos shoes, and his watch.

I went home, and Flo was home early from San Raphael, so she and I went back to the hospital. They had taken him for an x-ray, outside on the gurney, up and down ramps, bumping him around, and while they were doing that, he needed some oxygen, but – again, they didn't have any! Unbelievable!

We found that he was now in shock, and there was no blood available because, – I still can not believe this – the Red Cross was closed from 12 to 2pm for lunch.

But the Doctor was at fault, too, he should have gotten it long before, and had it going already. Now he ordered some Dextran, a volume expander, but the hospital, again, didn't have any. That is to say, they had 500cc, but since the Doctor ordered 1,000cc, they didn't give him any! Just unbelieveable!

Some one there went to the town pharmacy to get some, but came back with another bag of five percent glucose. I said I would give him some blood, as I am a universal donor, but they didn't have what was needed to type and cross-match. When they finally got that, Flo and I stood out in the hallway waiting while they took a young man first to match, and while we were waiting – Maizamo died! And they call this a hospital! He died from neglect and incompetence, nothing else! Just unbelievable!!

Then, the wailing and crying began. Some of Flo's students were there, all his friends, and they were all wailing and crying. His parents were there, and his mother was throwing herself around, and screaming while they tried to put her into the car. So sad! We went to see the family yesterday, and instead of being a witness for the Lord, and the fact that we will see him again, she was still screaming and wailing. What a culture. As Christians we should not follow a culture that has no hope.

October 29, 1988

I must write this to finish the sad story of our young Pastor Maizamo. Today was his funeral. It was to be in his little stick church that Flo and I had bought for him, but by the time we arrived, there were already far too many people to fit into it.

Then, they said it would be down the road about two miles farther, at a big church. About then, I heard all this screaming, and a pick-up bringing the casket, came roaring by, with a whole mob of screaming young women running after it. They were throwing their dresses up over their heads, and generally acting like demented people.

I had taken my car, and Flo drove her Rocky, both filled to the max with people. We had to cross two rivers, and my car hit bottom on the first one, so on the next, I had every body get out and walk, while I drove across. Less weight helped.

When we got to the bigger church, there was a huge crowd, so we decided to wait outside, and let all the others go in. It was loud pandemonium inside, with screaming, wailing, and lots of crazy activities. To me, it looked like nothing less than demon possession. They sure didn't behave like Christians who know they will see him again. It was so loud and wild inside that they couldn't even hear the service. They must have carried out ten fainting women at different times. I thought that one of them was going to fall down the steps, and take the men helping her, along with her. One woman was wallowing in the dirt of the road in her new dress, screaming and crying out his name. It was really awful! We will miss him very much.

November 4, 1988

Skip's pastor from the church in New York is here, along with his wife, and two nurses. The pastor is also Darlynn's father. I've talked to them about the clinic, and I guess we will just close it while I am gone for two months, but we will pay the workers to keep them.

Kathy and Alice received a letter from their pastor telling them that Pastor Cebien must sever his connections with Grace Church (does that include me?) or they will have to leave him and his work. They told the girls that John MacArthur is a heretic! I know that is something he definitely is not.

Dr. Bibiana had to leave and go back to her church in Venezuela, and she is working toward coming back, hopefully in April or May.

We've had a terrible rat problem at Babiole Clinic. I opened a drawer, and there was a whole family of baby rats in a nest. I finally bought some poison as they were eating everything, and making an awful mess.

Dr. Benson is here right now to visit Flo. He's signed Dr. Bibiana up to be a part of Medical Ambassadors, and now they're talking about hiring Dorléon. I pray that he will be wise enough to see any pitfalls. He is looking for a wife now – Francoise?

Last night, we had the biggest tarantula I have ever seen. He was as big as my hand; he covered the whole 12 inch tile on the floor. We finally had to call the yard man to come in and kill it. I hated to do it, but he was going all over the house.

Today we went to La Brié for a clinic. My little car crossed the rivers just fine, and Dr. Benson and a friend followed behind me in his little Mazda. We were all working in the clinic, when they came carrying a man who had accidentally chopped his foot with a big ax. How fortunate for him that there (in God's providence) just happened to be a surgeon there that day, who sewed him up. We were really glad that Dr. Benson was there, as we couldn't have done what he did. We were finished by 11:30am – incredible! Many hands really DO make light work.

November 5, 1988

Another big tarantula right on the floor next to my chair! Again, the electricity was off, and we were sitting in the semi-darkness of some candles. I turned my flashlight on him, and he turned around, and in typical tarantula fashion, went out the door, across the porch, and over the edge into the darkness, Oh! My shattered nerves!

November 6, 1988

I made an appointment to talk to Pastor Cebien today. It reminded me of the time I got the letter from him that surprised me so. He surprised me today with his openness, and when he talks to me like he did today, I find myself ready to do anything for him – well, almost. He just tries SO hard to make his big dreams come true, but he just never quite makes it; but he never gives up, either.

Listening to him yesterday as he talked to Flo and me about what his new school was, and what he is teaching, it sounded really good. Then, when he started talking about the revival he's having in his church, and what he was preaching on, I got enthused again.

Tonight we all went to his church, and he and Kathy and Alice sang, and it was beautiful! I was surprised that I understood most of the words of the songs, and his sermon. That's encouraging! *Thank You, Lord.*

November 8, 1988

I started figuring up my payroll for Morne Rouge clinic, and I keep saying that if I have to make it up out of my pocket, I just can't feel that it's the Lord's work. I am going to pay them tomorrow, as it will be the last clinic there until I come back in January of '89. I owed them forty-eight dollars, and I had fifty-five. Then I counted the Haitian money and I had another eight dollars which gave me sixty-three. I had forgotten about Ronnie, and he gets five dollars. When I added that, it was sixty-three dollars. Exactly what I needed! Praise the Lord – He wants me to stay, and keep on keeping on.

November 13, 1988

Tragedy after tragedy! Today was a usual Sunday – I listened to a tape of John's, and regretted that I hadn't asked Pastor Cebien to stop by and take me to church with him. There are two black ladies from Simi Valley in California, here visiting him, and I loaned him my car as he was using a rented one, and it was costing him too much money.

He had a great service where he explained the Gospel, and people who had thought they were saved, but now realized they weren't, came forward. There were fourteen people who came forward to trust Jesus. Pastor was thrilled by it, and was praising the Lord.

On the way back to Morne Rouge, at the place where Maizamo was hit, two big busses, were going into Cap-Haitien. On this two lane road one was trying to pass the other. He then sideswiped the bus, and sent him careening into Pastor Cebien – head on!

It was a terrible, terrible crash, but God protected and preserved the lives of everyone in my car! Pastor Cebien was hurt the worst, but he got out of the car immediately to help the women, and the three men in the back seat. Pastor Cebien had a big bump on his forehead, and it was bleeding. His nose was split, and his mouth was cut by his teeth. His right hand is hurt, especially his thumb. He probably has a broken rib, and he can't put any weight on his left leg as his knee hit the dashboard. He said he thought he was going to die.

The women, and Pastor were covered with tiny shards of glass, and one of the women had some facial lacerations. She also had a wrenched back, a four inch gash next to her knee, and cuts and scrapes here and there. The other woman had a big bump above her eye, a sprained ankle, plus cuts inside her mouth from the braces on her teeth. One of the Pastors in the back seat had a big 'X' gash to the bone on his forehead, and the other two Pastors were okay, with only cuts and bruises, thank God!

Two men were thrown off the top of the bus when it hit my car, and were killed on impact with the highway. The other bus that caused the accident, just kept going, on into town to the police station for protection. Three more people have died since the accident, which makes a total of five dead. It's hard to understand how people were killed, but when you look at my car, which was totaled; it's harder to understand how anyone lived!

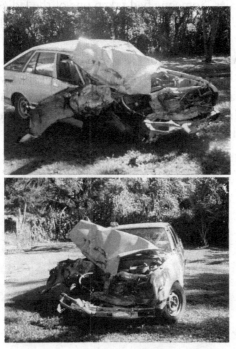

Ti-Limo after the crash

The engine was pushed up to the dashboard, and the hood is buckled up in the air. There is hardly any room at all in the front seat, and Pastor Cebien is all long legs.

The spot where Pastor's knee hit the dash is shattered. Somehow, all the papers for the car disappeared; I had put them in the glove box the night before, but, now they are gone. They said the battery was shattered. I hope and pray that the insurance you are forced to buy here, might cover at least some of the damage. Some say they will replace my car, or at least I might get some money out of it. I still owe twenty-five hundred dollars on it, which I will still have to pay, even though I now have nothing to show for the money.

It's the Lord's car, as everything I have is His. He knows my needs and has promised to supply them. I am just SO thankful that none of those in my car were killed, and I have to say, I am glad I was not in it, too. The car can be replaced, the people cannot!

Kathy and Alice just 'happened' to be right where it happened, at another missionary's house, and Dr. Harry just 'happened' to be at OMS to sew up the ladies. Someone had taken one of the ladies to the hospital on a tap-tap, so Flo and I rushed there to rescue her, and take her to Doctor Harry.

Kathy and Alice took Pastor Cebien to Flo's, and she took care of him, while I went with Kathy and Alice to take care of the two women. They were afraid to stay wherever they had been staying, and asked me to stay the night with them at the Hotel Mont Jolie, so I did. They took the next plane home, and I wonder if they will ever come back.

January 12, 1989 Back in Haiti

I have been gone from Haiti for two months, since the fifteenth of November,'88, and I arrived back in Haiti on Tuesday, the tenth of this month.

My first stop was New York to be part of a mission's conference at New Life Bible Church, for a week. Darlynn's dad is the Pastor, and they have the clinic at Babiole. Skip was also a part of it.

I had to speak for five minutes at every meeting, and that with no preparation ahead of time. The Lord was good, and He filled my mouth every session with His word.

When the conference was over, Skip and I went by car to Maryland, and stayed a week with my daughter Kathy and her husband Tony, and had Thanksgiving with them. On the twenty-eighth of November, I flew to California to be at Grace Church for the Outreach meeting on the thirtieth. My mom had been there visiting her sister in Burbank for two weeks, so on Sunday, we drove back to Tonopah. Then,I drove back to California on Tuesday for meetings with the Outreach Department at Grace Church.

On Wednesday, the seventh of December, I had a two hour meeting with four of the Outreach elders. One hour was about Pastor Cebien and Haiti, and the other was about Skip, as to any future plans. They told me that they would have a meeting to discuss it all, pray about it, and make a decision as to whether they felt I was eligible to re-marry.

I was baptized by John at Grace on the first day of this New Year. It was a wonderful, and terrible experience. I was so happy to have John baptize me, but the water was freezing COLD! They usually have it warm, but the heater wasn't working, (shades of Haiti) and when I walked out into it, in front of Maybe 1,500 people, the cold literally took my breath away, and I forgot everything I was going to say.

I went back to Tonopah, and on the ninth I flew to West Palm Beach, Florida, to fly back to Haiti on the tenth on Missionary Flights International's wonderful old DC-3, which pretty well brings this up to date again.

The elders at Grace called on the fourth to tell us that they didn't see any reason why Skip and I couldn't marry. I was surprised. I was so sure they would say no, and then Skip would have to give it up, and I could go on with my life. But, now, I don't know how this will work out. I'm still a little unsure. If I could be sure that it is the Lord's will for both of us, I would feel happy about it, but I felt that I needed to come back to Haiti for the next six months at least.

Pastor Cebien looks so thin and hollow eyed since the accident, but he is recovering, I'm just so thankful that the Lord spared him!

I went to Babiole clinic this morning to get it ready for a clinic on Tuesday, only to find that while I was gone, a truck had taken a short-cut through the yard. He had driven over the cesspool, caved in the top, and then, the truck had partially fallen in. Now, I have a gaping hole, lined with cement blocks, right where all 130 kids who will come on Tuesday, can fall into it.

Also, the men from the water department happened along just as I was leaving, and I told them, we had no water. They turned it on, and when they did, it sprayed up from a broken pipe outside. Someone had broken it, and then stolen the pipe from there to the house. The pipe from the house also has a big hole in it, as well, so they turned the water off again.

Then I went to the airport to pick up our mail, and the Customs officer told me that I had to go to the Commerce Department for a paper of some kind, because of all that I have had shipped in. I didn't know that I had any more coming in than anyone else, but it seems that I must pay in order to give it to the Haitians! They will 'out-greedy' themselves one day. Oh, well, the Lord knows what life is like here in this desperate place! He never said it would be easy, and sometimes I'm inclined to forget that I am engaged in an all out war! So, it's back to my Commander-In-chief for some more courage and endurance needed for the battle. The victory is ours, thanks be to Christ, who always causes us to triumph! Amen!

J.B.Phillips translation on Romans 5:3-5 ". . . . we can be full of joy here and now, even in our trials and troubles. Taken in the right spirit, (our response) these very things will give us patient endurance; this in turn will develop a mature character, and a character of this sort produces a steady hope that will never disappoint us."

I can understand why Paul could "rejoice in suffering, why James could "welcome trials as friends," and why Peter did "not think it strange, in the testing of your faith." All of these pressures and difficulties, have ultimate positive ends, and result in "praise, honor, and glory to Christ." The trials cannot steal our joy when we know that our God is sovereign; if we yield to the Spirit, we will not be overtaken by the difficulty.

January 17, 1989

A general strike in protest of President Avril today was responsible for canceling the opening of Babiole clinic again. There were no tap-taps, so I had no workers.

We didn't think that the MFI plane would come today, even though we were hoping they would, so poor Kathy here could get out to a Doctor. She fell last Saturday, and broke four bones in her left foot. She had Dr. Harry and Dr. Hall at OMS x-ray it, and their advice was – if she wanted to walk on it again, she should go to her Doctor in the States, and have it set properly. So – one week after we all got back, she and Alice left again for Pennsylvania. It's so interesting to see how the Lord works in all our lives. Pastor Cebien is hurt in an accident, my car is totaled, Kathy breaks her foot, and Alice has to leave again to help Kathy.

I received a very disturbing letter from a young woman at Grace Church, that I don't even really know. The Sunday I was there, she came up and told me who she was, and asked if she could write to me. I just thought she was one who was awed by us 'super-spiritual' missionaries, and said, "Sure."

She's written to me twice now. I answered her tonight, and I pray that it will help her. She was filled with fear and insecurity. I also advised her to seek some help from one of Grace's counselors. I pray that God will use the letter – I filled it with His Word, as I know mine is powerless. I also got my prayer letter done, and I hope I can get it out soon.

January 19, 1989

Opening day again at Babiole, and we only had about fifty kids. But out of that fifty, I had four, two and three month old babies, who only weighed five pounds each. One of them, whose mother was sick, and very anemic, had never had anything but tea and flour water in his entire life! No protein or glucose at all. She didn't have enough money to even buy him a baby bottle, I guess they spooned it into his mouth. I gave her $1.20 to buy a baby bottle, and I gave her some formula and some baby cereal. I should have taken a picture of him to send to the Ladies Bible Study in Tonopah, as I know they would send some food.

Another skinny baby boy had a mother who didn't want to feed him, I don't know why, or why she brought him here. So sad – poor little thing!

One little boy came with arms like sticks, little pointed chin, and huge sunken eyes. My guess was, he might have AIDS. He has the continuous diarrhea and large nodes in three places. I felt like I had to try something, so I put him on TB meds, as he may also have TB, and gave him lots of vitamins and food. I hope he will improve.

Pastor Cebien went to a funeral yesterday afternoon, and one of his students had a bad accident in a car on her way back home. Lange told me tonight that he saw the accident, and said the girl's car took off and flew!

Well, I went to the hospital with Pastor Cebien, and we waited for about four hours, again, while all they did for her was an x-ray. Finally, at 10pm, we went home, and after he ate something, he went back, put her in his car, and took her to Morne Rouge, where she is now an 'inpatient' in his 'hospital.' Her cervical vertebrae were fractured, and he has put her neck in a cast supported by two tooth brushes! He says she is much better, and asked me to go and check on her over the weekend while he goes to do a 'class repair job' on a church roof in the mountains, and I said, "Of course."

January 25, 1989

Well, poor Betty is having lots of pain, but she's wearing a cervical collar, and seems to be doing OK.

Yesterday, on our way to town, Flo and I saw something very sad; two men carrying a tiny coffin, with no one following it at all. What a commentary on the value of life in this country. Usually, there is a whole family following. Poor little baby- but then, it's far better off than those poor little ones who live – only to struggle all their lives with hunger, disease, ignorance and poverty. That baby is in the loving arms of Jesus.

I had only two patients today at Morne Rouge. I don't know why. I came home, did some washing, only to have five or six pair of underwear stolen off the backyard clothes line. I had washed today because I was running out – now I'm really out!

I just finished reading Dave Hunt's latest book; "America, The Sorcerer's New Apprentice." I'm really beginning to see where my Kathy and Tony are coming from. It's hard to believe that intelligent, educated people would fall for the very same lie that Satan told Eve in the Garden. It's incredible! Sorcery, witchcraft, and people believing they can become Gods – all being brought to them wrapped in a package labeled 'science, psychology, and nature.' We really are a nation of witless sheep, being led right onto the broad road marked 'Heaven', but leading straight to the Pit!

How I praise God – the only Creator of everything, that He has chosen me before the world began; to redeem me, sanctify me, and use me for His glory, and Eternity is mine – with Him! Amen!

January 29, 1989

I'm waiting for 8am when Skip is to call me. I seem to have 'tunnel syndrome' again. Both clinics are way down, no money, people to be paid, and no car. All of these things on my mind with Skip constantly pressing me as to when will we get married, while nagging at the back of my mind is the question, *'Do I really want to get married?'* I'm not sure I want to be a wife again, not sure I want to leave Haiti, and not sure I want to stay in Haiti. I seem to be in some kind of limbo.

No response from Pastor Cebien about my suggestion that we start our clinic days with Scripture and prayer together – I just feel like I'm accomplishing nothing here. Am I just here for Henri, Jonas, Ronnie, and all those whose need is for money only? Is that all I can do here? Hand out money? And right now, I can't even do that, since I don't have any!

I went down for Skip's phone call, and only succeeded in demoralizing and depressing him. I need someone with strength, to give me a dose of spiritual encouragement.

I picked up C.S. Lewis' Screwtape Letters, and read this; "He (Christ) is prepared to do a little over-riding at the beginning. He will set them off with communications of His presence, which, though faint, seem great to them with emotional sweetness, and easy conquest over temptation. But He never allows this state of affairs to last long. Sooner or later He withdraws, if not in fact, at least from their conscious experience, all those supports and incentives. He leaves the creature to stand up on it's own legs – to carry out from the will alone duties which have lost all relish. It is during such trough periods, (in the law of undulation) much more than during the peak periods, that it is growing into the sort of creature He wants it to be. Hence, the prayers offered in the state of dryness are those which please Him best . . . . He wants them to learn to walk, and must therefore take away His hand; and if only the will to walk is real, there He is pleased even with their stumbles. Do not be deceived, Wormwood. Our cause is never more in danger than when a human, no longer desiring, but still intending, to do our Enemy's will, looks around upon a universe from which every trace of Him seems to have vanished, and asks why he has been forsaken, and still obeys."

I seem to be in a very deep trough at present, one from which all supports have been withdrawn. I am indeed 'dry' but my desire is to be faithful; to keep on keeping on, knowing that He will again bring me to a 'peak' where the sun will be shining, with the blessings showering down again. Praise His name – He is my Lord, and my desire is to please Him by being obedient.

January 31, 1989

My little boat is rolled over by the waves that buffet it, yet I know He won't let it go under. Today, a letter – two letters- one from Dr. Bibiana to Dr. Benson, and one from Dr. Benson to Bibiana. I had written to Bibiana several weeks ago, that she didn't need to feel obligated to work in my clinics, as she had said that she was uncomfortable with kids, and that she preferred Flo's remote clinics. I understand this, and told her that whatever God puts on her heart to do, was what I hoped she would do. She said some of this in her letter to Dr. Benson and Medical Ambassadors. His reply was stuffy and full of clichés like, "I am your friend," and, "be sure all your money is sent to Medical Ambassadors," and then this, " I would like to mention that there is a clinic, formerly run by Diana, (whom Dr. Bibiana doesn't even know.) She came back to the U.S., about a year ago, to not return to Haiti. It would not be satisfactory for you to work at this clinic under the authority of the people who own the clinic. They are not the type of people we should be working with."

The arrogant audacity of this hypocritical man! He apologized to me, and then stabs me in the back with this! Dr. Bibiana wouldn't even be in Haiti if it weren't for me, but this seems to be conveniently forgotten.

And Flo! When I got angry, after reading this – she defended Dr. Benson on the grounds that, "they (the people who owned the clinic) were obnoxious!" He was talking about Darlynne's dad and mom, who were very excited to be going to see their daughter and her clinic in Haiti. Unfortunately, they were sitting next to Dr. Benson on the plane, but didn't know who he was at all. He was so annoyed by their high spirits and joyful noise that he seems to forget – along with Flo – that Bibiana came to Haiti in the first place because I wrote to her. Now, it's like they're waving the red flag in my face, and taunting me with, " Ha ha, she's ours now, and you can't have her!" And stupid me, I rose right to the bait. Now, I keep thinking of I Corinthians 13:".Love will hardly even notice when others do it wrong." The verse is speaking of 'agape' love. Well, I must confess to not only noticing it, but getting angry about it. I even wrote a quick letter to Dr. Bibiana, and mailed it. That man will never change. *"Forgive me, Lord."*

I found Pastor Cebien, and told him about it, and he suggested the verse of Paul's about, "When I was a child, I thought as a child, spoke as a child, etc. . ." for Dr. Benson. He also said he had another dream! Bad one, he said, and he would tell me about it tomorrow.

February 4, 1989

The unrest here is intensifying with the advent of Mardi Gras. Monday through Friday are supposed to be strike days. I don't know whether to try to have clinics or not. I was told that during Mardi Gras, people have the right to be on the streets, with the blessing of the Army, so going to town, or driving anywhere could be risky.

I have already had several experiences with this when I was with Pastor Cebien, and then again when I was driving Flo's Rocky. We were nearly stopped on our way down from Pastor Dorléon's church one Sunday.

On the way down the mountain, a whole group of people, some of them greased black with oranges for eyes – tried to spread across the road to stop us. I said, "Roll up the windows." We slowly went through, but it's frightening because you never know what they want, or what they might do. Usually, nothing happens, for which I thank the Lord, but there is always the potential for violence.

Then, there is our neighbor's puppy. He is chained up, crying continuously, so pitifully – all day long! When I asked why, they told me he had eaten a baby turkey. They called him a thief, and were punishing him. My answer was, "He's hungry! Feed him!"

Their answer was, "We have nothing to give him." I took him food three times today, and he literally inhales it.

The puppy's cries finally got to me so bad, that I clapped my hands over my ears, and cried. I just hate it – my stomach just churns all day long, hearing him cry. I think if any thing will drive me out of Haiti, it will be my inability to watch and hear their cruelty to helpless animals. I saw a puppy get hit by the car behind me in town- they don't even try to miss them – and I almost threw up. I have seen roosters hanging by their necks in trees as a voodoo sacrifice. I saw a man one day, walking along the side of the road, with a little cat hanging by its' neck from his hand. I saw a cow, trying to get out from under the front of a big bus, after the bus had hit it. Every day, somewhere, I hear the cries of dogs that have been hurt. It's a brutal place, and I hate that part of it.

But then, I guess when humans have to struggle just to survive, why should they be concerned about the suffering of an animal, when their lives are not much better than an animals' life.

I'm so glad God says that He cares about the animals. They were created by Him, and He has no pleasure in their pain, especially at the cruel hands of fallen man. I feel like I'm coming apart. I just want to sit and cry.

"A righteous man cares for the needs of his animals, but the kindest acts of the wicked are cruel." Proverbs 12:10

February 5, 1989

Today was a wonderful rest. I sat all day doing counted cross-stitch, and listened to some tapes of Grace Church services, plus one of John's sermons in Matthew. A dear friend at Grace Church sent the tapes to me, and they are a real blessing. I almost – not quite, but almost – feel like I've been sitting there in the church with that big crowd of believers. It was wonderful! I really thank the Lord for his thoughtfulness in taping them and sending them to me.

Here's a funny excerpt from C.S.Lewis' Screwtape Letters:

"It is in some ways more troublesome to track and swat an elusive wasp, than to shoot at close range a wild elephant. But the elephant is more troublesome if you miss."

February 6, 1989

When I arrived at Morne Rouge clinic this morning, I learned that one of the orphans at Morne Rouge had been hit by a camion (big bus) and was killed instantly. It happened about 7:30 last night, just beyond the Davis' driveway. Pastor Néonce went and got Pastor Cebien, so he was there at the clinic this morning.

He said to me, "Today is your day to come back with me to my seminar, and teach my students how to give a shot."

He went to town to get a coffin made for the boy who was killed, and on his way back, he stopped and picked me up, and we went back to the seminar.

I had thought it was a seminar on Epilepsy, but it turned out that his students were teaching the villagers about a variety of health topics. I gave my very first class: 'How to give a shot.' They loved practicing giving shots to an orange with water. After the class, we all had lunch – good Haitian food, and then most of the girls headed to the river to 'freshen up.' When they came back, Pastor Néonce gave a really good talk on being 'servants' – very needful!

I had to leave after that as I wanted to get home before dark. I ran into a huge group of Mardi Gras folks at Limbé. They were up ahead of me, surrounding a camion, so I took the side road by the hospital and went around behind them. I have to admit it was a bit scary, but there weren't any more the rest of the way – praise the Lord!

They say there will be a demonstration tomorrow at 10am. I still plan on having clinic, but I probably won't have many patients. I only had three at Morne Rouge today. I made six dollars, and it cost me twenty-one to pay the helpers. I sent Ronnie with the six dollars to buy some medicine.

I am reading a book about the history of missions. It is called From Jerusalem to Irian Jaya. In the chapter on medical missionaries is a great illustration of the problem one faces in communicating instructions on taking medicine properly to illiterate people. It reads; "On one occasion, they (the missionaries) left medicine with a mother for her sick child, and instructed her to give a dose each morning when the rooster crowed. When they returned some days later and inquired about the child, the mother replied, "My boy is fine now, but the rooster died!"

More and more I realize how much a foreigner I am in this place, but I love it anyway.

February 7, 1989

We had only about 28 patients this morning at Babiole, and we were finished by 9:30. I then went to the airport with Flo on that terrible back road as they were burning tires on the main road. Today is both Mardi Gras, AND the anniversary of the revolution, so they were really getting wild.

The plane was late, and on the way home, we had a flat tire, but because the road is so rough, Flo didn't realize it was flat until we were back on the main road, and by then, it was destroyed. And, it was a new one!

This evening, I had taken my shower, put on clean clothes, eaten my dinner, and I was beginning to work on my counted cross-stitch, when someone came to the door. I supposed it was someone wanting money, so I asked out the window who he was. I heard, "Pastor Cebien and Mme. Néonce."

Pastor Cebien needed some help with transportation to get people down off of the mountain after a church service. So – since I have Kathy and Alice's truck while they are gone, I went to help him. When I got to the church, I loaded up thirteen girls, and he loaded his machine and we started down the mountain again. He was following me, and I was glad because I was so loaded it was hard to steer or stop.

When we got back to Morne Rouge, they had a party. Pastor Cebien picked up his accordion, and made up funny jingles about some of his students, and they just loved it! His charisma is really something. You just can't help but love him – or hate him – which, I guess some do. Maybe someday I'll get used to him, or really understand him. I really need for God to tell me whether I should continue on with this man.

The latest is, he wants me to teach English to his students! I've never taught anything – and I am not a teacher, yet because he asks me, I hear myself say, "Of course, I will." I don't believe it.

Sometimes, I'm afraid that missionaries end up doing things they're not really qualified to do. But I think this glorifies the Lord, because He must give the enabling. First – I'm a doctor, and now, an English teacher! What next – I'm afraid to think about what he may think of for me to do. Whatever it might be, I just pray that I will be able to do it joyfully, and as unto the Lord, because without His enabling, I can do nothing.

February 12, 1989

Today, Pastor Néonce came by and asked me to take the coffin for the orphan that was killed, to the hospital. Again, since I had their truck, what could I say? It sure wouldn't fit in his car! So, I took it and them, to the hospital. Then, I had to retrace my steps at 2pm to take the coffin (now with a body in it,) back to the church at Morne Rouge. I decided to stay for the funeral, and it began very quietly – no screaming, only the sobbing of the little boy's classmates.

Pastor Cebien had let the church for a second funeral however, and they brought the coffin in, right in the middle of our service, and it was accompanied by all the screaming and writhing women, so I left. Pastor Cebien had been in Port, but he made it back for the funeral.

February 13, 1989

We had over 20 patients today, and Fre'Louis does very well getting two dollars from nearly all of them. I was thinking today I had made enough to pay everyone, and still have a bit over to buy medicine – when Felix showed up. He's a thirteen year old street kid, with diabetes, and no family, so I feel like I have to help him if I can. He's really a nice kid, but he never fails to show up at a bad time.

Today, after clinic, I made two trips to Pastor Cebien's new church-school building with benches, a pulpit, and a chair for Pastor Cebien; so Flo could have her class in his new building. He tells me I even have an office there as his 'secretary', and since I'm going to teach an English class, I think I should be promoted to Vice President of the school, at least! That's sort of on a par with doubling my salary – you know 0x0= ? Right! Praise the Lord!

Tomorrow Kathy and Alice will be back again. I have been able to use their truck while they were gone, but just the other day, Ronnie got a car! It's not really his, but he can use it, so he will drive me back and forth to Morne Rouge. Isn't the Lord GOOD! It just thrills me to see the Lord work, His timing is always perfect! Always!

February 14, 1989

There are so many things going through my mind tonight. I got the most discouraging letter from my mom today – really didn't need that, but then I got two letters and a valentine from Skip. In one of his letters was this wonderful verse. "Even to your old age and gray hairs, I am He. I am He who will sustain you. I have made you, and I will carry you. I will sustain you, and I will rescue you." Isaiah 46:4 NIV

I know that it was the Lord who was speaking to me from His word, and through His obedient servant. How I needed that sweet word of encouragement from Him. With no car, no money, and this terrible letter from my mom, plus Pastor Cebien left today on the plane that brought Kathy and Alice back. He had some word that his son was having a problem with his eyes, so he felt he had to go and take care of it. He said he'd be back in a week, but his one week frequently grows into two or three. That means I'll probably have his patients as well as mine tomorrow. It just always seems so much harder when he is gone.

I got some money today from Tonopah, but by the time I pay all my bills I won't have much left to help anyone else. Money seems to be becoming somewhat of a problem – or should I say, the lack of it, but I know my Provider knows, and He knows that I cannot help these poor brothers and sisters in Christ, unless He sends the money to do it.

It is impossible for those in comfortable homes, with good food on the table every day, to feel the desperation of a Haitian mother laying her feverish baby on a floor, made mud by rain, to sleep. She has no hope of any money to buy food or medicine for her baby. No food for herself or her other children who have gone to sleep hungry. She loves the Lord, and she prays, "Oh, Lord, please send me just some food for my children, and then she comes, reduced to begging, and asks me if I can help her. I praise God that He has used me to help them, and answer their prayer for help.

In my clinic, I sit and look at the apathetic, edematous face of a little child dying of kwashiorkor. Every once in awhile his eyelids very slowly lift and blink. As I examine him, he shows no interest, and no resistance to my touch. His hands look like balloons with fingers, and his lower legs and feet are worse. Because of the edema, at first glance one might think he is chubby, but on closer inspection – I raise up his shirt to disclose prominent ribs, and push up his sleeve to show me an upper arm that my fingers can wrap around twice!

His hair is a pale brackish yellow-red color, which means – he is getting no protein. His heart rate is erratic – he is slowly dying, even as I examine him.

His mother has died – a familiar story – and his aunt is caring for him. She has numerous children of her own who must be fed, and this three year old is at the end of the food line. He desperately needs food – mainly protein - the body building essential for every child, and I have no milk today to give to him. I give him what I have, but with a breaking heart, I watch him being carried out, and I wonder if he will live for me to see him again next week.

I think of Jesus, compassionate Savior, who took the children up in His arms and blessed them, and my heart sends up a prayer for this small boy, that the Lord will do what I can't do, and heal him for His glory. I am here because Jesus loves these little children, and His command was to GO!

As far as progress- how does one measure progress by God's measuring rod? What does progress mean in God's economy? He really doesn't ask to see our record of how much we have accomplished – numbers are not the issue – faithfulness is!

February 17, 1989

Tomorrow is the BIG day for Scott and Faith, two of our missionary friends. It's their wedding day! I am so happy for them. To think that they have never even kissed each other, now that's purity! How strange that must seem to the world. It's too bad that more Christian young people don't follow this example. What a beautiful gift they have to give to each other. I really admire them, and I know He will bless this union.

Well, things seem to be heating up on the political scene here in Haiti. We heard of trouble, shooting, and riots today in Fort Liberty, which is east of Cap-Haitien, and also in Saint Mark, Gonaieves, and Port au Paix. Frances and her girls went – alone - today to Port au Paix. I hope they'll be able to get back home again. Lange was here this evening, and he was talking about Saint Mark – the schools are supposed to be closed, but there were some there that were open. They (I'm not real sure who 'they' are) went to the school, took the kids outside, roughed them up a bit, tore their uniforms, and sent them home. You really have to be brave to frighten and attack children!

I'm about ready to leave, and let them have this place. Maybe my mom's right after all, maybe God is trying to tell me something. Maybe I should leave. I wonder if Pastor Cebien will have a problem getting back. I sit and think – could I leave knowing I might never see him again, or Kathy and Alice, or Sandy, or all of these precious brothers and sisters in Christ here.

I really don't think I'd want to come back married. I don't know why exactly, but I just feel that Skip and I would have a new and different ministry if we marry.

I cleaned my room thoroughly today. I even washed my bedspread and curtains, and cleaned my screens. Everything was so nice and clean, but I sure was dirty when I finished. I just got it all off of the clothesline before the rain came, and then got my shower before the electricity went off. Praise the Lord, He is so good to me!

Heard there is to be another strike on Monday. Pastor Cebien returned one week after he left, and with a new generator for his new church at Champin!

February 23, 1989

The plane came today with Richard, the 'begger', and Flo got over 300 pounds of powdered milk, and boxes of medicines.

Today at Babiole clinic, after about an hour, I began to be aware of a rumble of voices outside, growing louder and louder. I tried to ignore it, but when all of my help began to disappear one by one, I asked Ronnie to please go out and see what was going on. He came back and said, "Well, Miss Pat, now you are a mother!"

Of course I said, "WHAT?" And then he told me that a little girl had been abandoned, and I would have to care for her. I said, "Oh, no, if I do that, the next thing I know, I will be an orphanage!"

The buzz outside continued, so I went out to look, and there she sat, all by herself.

I had seen this child a week ago, and had sent her to Dr. Harry, because she could not walk or talk, and she was two years old. She could sit up, but her legs were slightly atrophied, and to me, she looked a bit microcephalic, and somewhat retarded, though she didn't have a dull look, but rather, her eyes were bright and lively. She was a sweet little thing, and would smile easily.

She was brought back today by her parents, and had been sitting on the bench between them when I was passing out numbers. She looked very well cared for, with little ear-rings in her ears; her skin, hair, and clothes were clean, and she had a bright red ribbon in her hair.

The dad had handed me the letter Dr Harry had written to me, which I read and handed back to him, telling him, I would read it again when he got inside. I can't imagine how desperate these parents must have been, because when they were almost inside, they just left her sitting there all alone.

Two of the ladies who work with me offered to take her home and care for her. These are Christian ladies who both have lots of kids of their own that they are struggling to feed. One lady is a widow, but she offered first. Then, the other offered as well. The first one has four children, one of whom has a bone problem, and needs a brace on one leg. Both she and her husband are working, but their kids sleep on a dirt floor, and they really have nothing. I told her I would help her buy food for the child. Poor little thing! She just sits and looks at you, bewildered.

Then, I had a return visit of a baby I've been seeing since it was a five pound newborn. The mother was sick and couldn't nurse it, which is usually a death sentence for a baby. Today, it weighed six pounds, but it is two months old! It is skinny, and lay wide awake sucking fiercely on it's fingers. When I asked how often the baby was fed, I was told four times a day, and four times a night. Not too bad.

When I asked how much was it fed each time, I was told, an ounce to an ounce and a half. Then, I asked if the baby was ready to stop after that amount, or if she would take more. She said, "Oh, she would take more, but I'm afraid I'll run out, and not have any more to feed her." How sad. Of course, I said, "Please, give this baby all she will take, and I will give you more as you need it. She needs the food, and is not sick, so she can take it."

"Oh, Lord, You see this tiny one that You alone have given the gift of life. Please help me to help her – for Your glory! Please bless the two workers for their example of Christian love – self sacrificing – in being willing to take this abandoned child to care for. Amen!

Later note: The mother of the abandoned child in my clinic came to our house about two weeks later and just wanted to see the child. We told her no, that it would be too traumatic for the child to see her mother, and then be left by her again; it wasn't fair to the child. We told her the child was being well cared for, and would stay where she was, at least for the present. If the mother wanted her back, and could assure us that the child would be taken care of, and NOT abandoned again, we would consider it. She finally said she wanted her back, and would not leave her again, so we arranged for the child to be returned.

The worker, who had been caring for her was able to get the child to stand up, and was working on helping her to speak as well. We only hope the mother will do the same. The worker said she would show the mother what she had been doing, and help her to do it as well, so maybe the good outcome of this will be a walking, talking child. Nothing is impossible with God!

February 27, 1989

I had my every other week Saturday phone call from Skip. It was rather disappointing in that instead of encouraging me to be faithful here, even without sight of progress his comment was, he can't see why I am really needed here.

Between him and my mom – the very two who should be encouraging me the most – I am beginning to really feel like a failure. I know I am right where God wants me to be for now, anyway. One day at a time, I'll walk behind my gentle Shepherd. I don't 'see' any accomplishments either, but one can only live a life before others – in a life time – not in just a year or two.

My mom says, she is tired of helping to support me, and I think Skip is as well. We'll see just how real his 'unconditional' love for me is.

It's true he is doing much more for the Lord in his jail ministry than I am in my clinics. I've told him that before. He's bringing lost men to a saving knowledge of the Lord almost every time he goes to the jail, and I think that is wonderful!

I pray that one day I will be released from this, but for now, I will strive to be faithful in the face of my 'Job's Comforters'.

March 12, 1989

It's a lovely Sunday – cool and beautiful, and quiet. There is a nurse from Skip's church in New York, whose name is Jerri, and she has come to stay for a year. She will take over Babiole as soon as she feels comfortable there alone, and I will concentrate on Mourne Rouge, at least for awhile, and then I may go home and marry Skip, if that is the Lord's will for us.

I listened to John's tape on Philippians 2:17 and 18 this morning, and was really blessed. Here are some choice gleanings from the tape – all on 'sacrifice = joy!'

Quote: "The level of joy is proportional to the level of sacrifice. It is not related to our human circumstances. It is joy in spite of, not because of. The greater the sacrifice, the greater the joy; the more supreme the offering, the greater the exhilaration. Your effectiveness as a Christian is directly related to one thing – the proximity in which you live in intimate fellowship with Christ. An abiding branch bears fruit."

My thoughts on it were – as John spoke about those sitting there listening, who had never experienced this spiritual joy, because they know nothing of sacrifice, I felt sorry for them, because what they don't realize, is that it only looks like a sacrifice, but when it is given, it in itself - becomes the joy. One can't know this though, until they have been willing to take up their cross – the sacrifice of their life- and then, what joy! It is only our great God who could cause this to be so. It is all of Him! Amen!

In thinking more, and praying more about what the Lord's will for my life might be after July, I have been wondering and comparing what the differences in my ministry might be. It might be that I would have a better ministry – more effective in use of my time, and people reached – if I married Skip, and went with him into a different ministry. It's a concern for prayer. I just have not been willing to even think in that direction yet, but I'm beginning to feel that I must be willing to change if that is what the Lord desires. Maybe, He has brought me here for a purpose that is accomplished now.

March 17, 1989

Last night I woke up about 1:45am, and I could hear the drums very close. I looked out the window in the dining room, and the sounds were coming from an area just across the field from us. I could hear their voices and see the fire as well. Too close! How sad to be a slave of Satan and his hosts of demons.

In this land of starving people, it's not surprising that the animals are starving as well. The poor little puppy of our neighbors is SO pitiful, and what really makes me angry is that she can afford to feed him! I'll just never understand the mentality of people who have NO concern for the suffering of any animal. That puppy is just skin and bones with two little eyes that she rolls in fear when I approach her. She is really a 'broken in spirit' little dog. When I stop to pet her, she makes little crying noises and scoots on her belly on the ground. I think I am the only human who has ever shown her any kindness. I have been feeding her, trying to save her, but I don't have enough to really help her.

Raoul, our yardman, has a little dog named Mickey. He has become a very nice and well behaved little guy. Mickey was so cute today. He has two little goat friends, who are usually tied in the field next to our house. During the day, he goes over to see them, and bark at them, to see if they will play with him.

Today, they weren't tied, their ropes were there, but they were dragging them. He went over to play, and after some nose touching, some agile leaps, and more fancy footwork, he got the rope of one of them in his teeth, and was pulling on it.

Now, if there's anything a goat hates, it's having his rope pulled, and there was some real objecting to this, much to the startled surprise of Mickey. It was so cute! It's so seldom one sees something pleasant here with animals, so I stood and watched them for quite a while – much to Flo's disgust, but what I was watching was priceless! Someday, all the animals will play together, Praise the Lord !

3/21 The puppy is putting on weight and looks much better.

March 22, 1989

Often on the Rock I tremble,
Faint of heart, and weak of knee;
But the mighty Rock of Ages
Never trembles under me.
Author Unknown

I wrote this in here a few days ago so I wouldn't lose it, never dreaming how appropriate it would be for today.

It was only 7am when I arrived at Morne Rouge for my clinic. I was met by Pastor Cebien who said to me, "You'd better hurry as there is a very sick baby inside."

I ran in, took one look at the baby lying in its mother's lap, and went to make some oral rehydration fluid for it. As I brought it back for the mother to give to the baby, I noticed she was shaking the baby and poking it - all with no response from the baby whatsoever. I got my stethoscope out, and listened; my worst fear was realized. It was already gone. Nothing would help it now.

I went and told Pastor Cebien. He came and listened, and agreed. I told him, he should tell her, though we both knew that she already knew.

He told her, and she began shrieking. The baby began to slide, and roll off of her lap. As she stiffened out on the bench, the baby began to roll down her legs, and I just caught it before it got to the floor. I picked it up, and laid it in the baby scale on the counter.

By now, the mother was rolling around on the dusty cement floor, screaming and crying; every person within earshot was standing at the door watching. There was no one with her but a poor, frightened little girl of about six or seven years old, so Pastor Cebien sent someone to find the dad.

They got the mother out of the treatment room, and then she began rolling all over the waiting room floor, shrieking and crying, "Amway!" (Help)

I began seeing three other babies who were waiting, as their mothers were all thoroughly frightened now for their babies.

My helpers began to arrive, and things began to settle down a bit. Then I noticed that the mother of the dead baby had left! Without the baby!

When the father arrived, people told him the baby was dead, and he was going to leave as well, without the body of the baby. Pastor Cebien ran after him, caught him, and brought him back to the clinic. He told others to keep him there, while he went and flagged down a pick-up truck who was passing on his way to town. Pastor told the dad to get in the back of the truck, gave him the body of the baby and told the driver to go!

They had left the body of the baby because, Pastor told me, they couldn't afford a funeral, and they thought I would pay for it. It has been a time of great pain, and I find myself longing for some strong arms of comfort.

Later that day, I went with Pastor Cebien into his 'inpatient' room where he was taking care of a boy who was just skin and bones. He had been burned quite a while back, but had survived that. Now, they said he couldn't eat, because of the sores in the corners of his mouth. Actually, I thought the sores were probably the result of vitamin deficiency because he wasn't eating. Pastor Cebien began to put some of his medicine in the boy's mouth, but it was so painful for the boy, that I just couldn't stay, and I had to leave.

I went out, flagged down a tap-tap, and went home. I cried a bit and prayed for the mother of the baby that died, the boy in such pain, and for me. I looked for the puppy to feed it. While I was looking for it, the little boy who owned the puppy, ran out and planted himself right in front of me saying, with a big grin on his face, "Oh, Miss Pat, the puppy died!"

Too much, too much today. How thankful I am for the comfort of the Lord Jesus! I am fighting so many things here. I really am beginning to feel that I must leave! Philippians 4:8 tells me what I have to do – think on the things that please and glorify Him; His strength is made perfect in my weakness. I can do all things through Christ who strengthens me. Amen!

I just tore yesterdays date off of my calendar, and here is the verse for this sad day: "He giveth power to the faint; and to them that have no might, He increaseth strength." Isaiah 40:29 KJV

He always knows our needs and supplies them all, as we need them. He is a great and wonderful, awesome God. What a blessing to serve Him!

I was talking to Ma'Louie today about doing 'nasty' jobs. She had offered to clean up the mess I had made making 'pomade soufre' (Vaseline mixed with sulfer powder for scabies.) I said there was no reason why I couldn't do it, no reason why she should have to do all the dirty jobs. I didn't have a broken arm, and didn't the Lord teach us that we are to be servants, and do for others? She gave me a Creole saying, then, "M'pa ginynin main l'or!" "I don't have hands of gold!" I love it!

April 2, 1989

Today, I became a god-mother, a 'marin'. It was Simone's baby's dedication day at church, and she asked me to be his god-mother. (I hope this doesn't mean that I have to take him home with me!) It was a nice, but long and hot service. His pretty white outfit I had bought for him was too small, so he wore a cute red outfit I had brought back for him in January. He is so cute!

Today, I am free of Babiole clinic. What a load off of my shoulders! I am so glad! Now, I can be at Mourne Rouge at least three, and maybe four days a week. I can use Pastor Cebien's students, and maybe save some money to buy meds with. Praise the Lord!

Al Mount is coming to Port-au-Prince on Tuesday, but isn't coming here until the tenth, and then only for the day.

Jerri, the nurse who has taken over Babiole clinic, has moved into her new house, and seems to be really happy to be there. She's a sweet girl, and so pretty. I have given her all the books for Babiole, but I need to get my suction machine, and ambu bags, and take them to Morne Rouge.

It is being impressed on me more and more that I am going to have to leave Haiti to survive! But I don't want to go home to be a house-wife in New York for two to three years until Skip can retire from Kodak. Maybe I can go home for a month in August, get married, and we could go on the Alaska Cruise with Grace Church. Then, I could come back here for maybe four months – go home for a couple of weeks in December or January – and come back here for another three months. Then I could go home to stay in April of 1990, and then Skip would retire in July. Sounds good to me! The Lord knows, but I have a feeling that this wouldn't be to Skip's liking at all.

Pastor Cebien says he would come after me if I left, but I know he wouldn't. He'd just solicit someone else. I'm hoping to begin my 'English Class' for him on Thursday afternoon. I have sat at the typewriter all week trying to work up the classes. I am up to lesson #5, but I may not be able to cover all the material in that time, so I won't do any more until I see how they go. I think it will be fun.

Flo has been sick for a few days, but seems to be better today.

Sandy came by and said he'd heard that there was another coup in the early hours of the morning, and that Avril was in prison. I hope we can find out tomorrow just what has happened.

April 4, 1989

Jerri's first day at Babiole went well, and I am so glad. The workers all seem to like her, though how anyone could NOT like her I don't know. She is so beautiful – inside and out – very sweet, always smiling or laughing, and so good to look at! She is learning the language very quickly as well.

In my clinic, I only had four kids, and made $9. That was yesterday. I didn't have a clinic today, as I had planned to take Flo to the airport, but due to more political upheaval, the airport was closed today, so MFI didn't come.

The woman I bought my car from got on my case today about my wrecked car that is still in a neighbor's front yard. Pastor Cebien keeps saying he is going to move it, but it's still there. She said he has to move the car this week! I had to agree with her that it has been there much too long, but he says he is waiting on the insurance company, and they're in Port-au-Prince. They said they want to see it before giving me any money.

I went to talk to Pastor to tell him what she said, and he said again, that he will move it.

4/5 He moved the car into his yard at Morne Rouge today.

April 9, 1989

Today was quiet, though yesterday afternoon they were up to their old tricks of burning tires and shooting off guns. I really don't know why, and most of them probably don't know why either. It just seems to be something exciting to do.

Last night, around mid-night, I was just dozing off, when I heard two shots, very close, and then they were followed by four more in quick succession. I lay there waiting to hear screaming, or something else to happen, and when nothing did, I rolled over and began to drift off to sleep again, Then again, in another place, farther away, there were another six shots. Again, followed by nothing – so I went to sleep, and this morning no one said anything about something happening, so I have no idea what was going on.

Poor Jerri is having a serious problem in her clinic at Babiole. Her staff is rebelling after she announced her changes; and there seems to be a ringleader. I think they're testing to see how far they can push. She sent me a note, and they want me to come to a meeting after my clinic on Tuesday. If I go, I will give them four Scriptures: Ephesians 5:21, Romans 13:1&2, Hebrews 13:17, and Titus 3:1. They all deal with the subject of submission to authority, and the fact that it is God who places people in authority, and when you choose to rebel against that authority, you are rebelling against God, and are putting yourself in a very dangerous position. This cannot be tolerated if they call themselves Christian – and they do. Twice, in a very short note, the ringleader wrote ' Si Dieu vlé' - if God wills. I will try to show them, by God's grace and the Holy Spirit – just exactly what it is that God does will – submission to authority.

My English class was to have begun at 2pm on Thursday at Champin. I walked over – took me about twenty-five minutes, but by 2:30, I still had no room to use and no blackboard, as Pastor Cebien had assured me I would have. Pastor Néonce was having a Bible School class in the room I was supposed to have, and nothing had been said to him about my class. I explained to Pastor Dorléon, that if I let this go, and tried to teach this way, it would never be better, but if I just went home, maybe just maybe, the message would be heard, that people need to do what they say they will do. It's called integrity.

I asked Pastor Dorléon to explain to the few who were there. They were angry that they had come, and it was inconvenient for them! I said, "Don't talk to me about inconvenient – I walked all the way here as I had no car."

I suggested they talk to Pastor Cebien, and I walked back home. Poor Ronnie, he was in the middle of both my problem, and Jerri's that day! I hoped that if Pastor Cebien was really concerned or interested, he would come by to talk to me about it, but he hasn't.

When I talked to Skip yesterday, I told him to call and see if the cruise to Alaska was booked. If it's not, we'll have our honeymoon studying and cruising. If it is booked, we'll go to Scotland – Lord willing.

April 22, 1989

Skip called this morning, and he's gotten the tickets for the Alaska Cruise, and we've also planned to go to Scotland first, sometime in July. Then, I'll plan to try and get my mother settled somewhere that she'll be happy. I'll go back to New York, and back to work in a hospital there until Skip retires. All of this - as the Lord wills.

I've been reading, and listening to many messages on marriage, and I am still dragging my feet! I just don't believe I will make a good wife. In fact, right now I don't believe I would make a good anything! What I thought was my ministry seems to suddenly be nonexistent.

The two new nurses are here with Flo now, after spending their first two weeks at the hospital in Limbé. They both seem very nice, and Flo seems quite happy with them. One plays the piano, and the other girl plays the flute. They play together, and it's very pretty music.

I have no English class, and I only see two or three kids on Monday and Wednesday. I believe the Lord is closing this door.

April 27, 1989

Things here just point more and more to my leaving, and that – soon. I'm not sure I will even stay until June. There just doesn't seem to be any reason for me to stay, at least that I can see. This morning I really feel it. My clinic at Morne Rouge is nearly one year old, and I never see more than ten kids each day. I have given up on Pastor Cebien, that is, in helping him directly, and my English class never materialized. Kathy and Alice will be teaching there next year, so I'm not really needed there either.

I'm waiting now on the elders at Grace Church to send me their decision on the letter I sent to them, giving them my plans as I see them now, to leave and marry Skip. I feel like I'm just occupying space here now. It's humiliating to go to my clinic, see three or four kids, and then come home and do counted cross-stitch, while everyone else is running around – so busy. I feel so utterly unnecessary and useless. No one needs me. It's a humbling experience trying to somehow justify my presence here to these two girls who've just arrived, and to everyone else, for that matter.

Again – I know the Lord didn't make a mistake in bringing me here, but it is finished here for me. I hope I have done what He wanted me to do while I was here. I don't feel that I have accomplished anything, but the Lord knows how He will judge on that, and they are not always the things that man judge's success or failure by. I have tried to be faithful and to please Him. His is the only judgment that really matters to me.

April 28, 1989

Last Monday, when I got off of the tap-tap from my clinic, I was met by a teary eyed, trembling Henri from Limbé. He told me that his wife had died in the hospital at 1am that morning. They had been together for twelve years (although they got married only last year – no money) I thank God that I have been able to help some of these poor, poor people here. It's a very fine line between helping them, and making them dependent on you, and when I could, I have given them jobs to do, so they can earn the money. It makes them feel better about taking the money, and I have given Henri some jobs to do; I even bought him a wheel-barrow so he could do other jobs as well. But, I know that there are a few who are regular 'takers', but some are also unable to work.

One is the annoying, raucous, persistent, toothless, skinny old man who told me one day, that Flo, unknowingly, I'm sure, had slammed the door in his face, and 'frappéd' his fingers in the door! I've been told that he probably drinks the money I give him. Today, I gave him some empty gallon jugs, and told him he could sell them for some money. He went away muttering, "Mesi mama, mesi mama"

Henri was back again today. Sometimes, he is a real trial. He has a speech impediment, and for me to understand Creole is difficult, and then when he talks, I really have a hard time understanding him. When he comes, he stands with his arms raised up braced on the side of the door, and with the heat and humidity, lack of soap and water, I have to stand about three feet back from the door, just to breathe. Today, he brought his daughter with him. I know the Lord loves him, and for that reason, I love him as well.

May 3, 1989

Today was a very bad day for our autos. I have been driving another missionary's Rocky while she is in the States. Flo's Rocky uses diesel gasoline, but Lois's uses regular gas. This morning I took Ronnie with me, and we went to the gas station to fill up Lois's Rocky. I drove right up to the diesel pump, (I was used to filling Flo's) and put $17.50 worth of diesel fuel in it.

I decided then, to go and get some beans, and as I was driving down the street, it began to cough and sputter. It suddenly hit me what I had done! I had just put diesel fuel in a gasoline engine! And it was NOT working! I managed to get back to the station, and they had to drain it all out. Then they filled it again, plus they charged me ten dollars for doing it.

I was so glad that I had Ronnie with me! I would never have been able to make them understand what I had done without him. He talked for me, so he really earned his five dollars for the day. It's OK again, but it took a lot of pumping the gas pedal to get it started, and to keep it going until all the diesel fuel was out of the lines.

Then- Flo's Rocky lost a rear wheel – it just came off, and went rolling down the street ahead of us, all by itself. The resultant drop to the pavement damaged the wheel and the axel, so her car is laid up for awhile. Maybe the Lord wants us ALL to go home!

One bright spot in my day, I received a very nice letter from John MacArthur, but I feel so ashamed – he thinks I'm really doing something – and here I sit!

May 5, 1989

I've been reading a biography of Isobel Kuhn, called <u>"One Vision Only"</u>, by Carolyn Canfield. It is another story of a brave missionary, a pioneer, who lived every moment of every day for the Lord. It makes me feel so ashamed. My tiny two year stint here has been a vacation in comparison. She was quite a lady, and died of cancer in her early fifties.

Here are a few gems I took from the book:

"The good things of life must never displace the best things!"
"The Spirit filled life is a daily grind."

In her small apartment that she fixed up for herself and her children at Wheaton, she said that she would often whisper to the Lord, "Thank Thee Lord, but don't let my heart get tied to it. Help me to remember it's just a tent, with the friendship of God and my friends upon it."

"If we send our roots down deep into a thing of earth, that very thing May set up spiritual decay in our being." How true!

I read a wonderful portion of Scripture today, and it's just one more that says God wants us to give to those in need. It's II Corinthians 9:12-15. I love it!

"This service that you perform is not only supplying the needs of God's people, but is also overflowing in many expressions of thanks to God. Because of the service by which you have proved yourselves, men will praise God for the obedience that accompanies your confession of the Gospel of Christ, and for your generosity in sharing with them and with everyone else. And in their prayers for you, their hearts will go out to you, because of the surpassing grace God has given you. Thanks be to God for His unspeakable gift!" LB Amen! And Amen!

And the really wonderful part is – God gets thanked for the same gift at least three times. First, by the one who has earned it; secondly, by me thanking Him for sending it, and for the one who sent it; and thirdly, by the poor person who receives it. And to think there are those who say it's wrong to give them money, especially when I know that I am ministering my Spirit given gift – that of giving.

May 11, 1989

I talked to Skip Tuesday evening after he had talked by phone to Al Mount for an hour. My letter hasn't been discussed yet by the elders, but the gist of the conversation was – wait – again! So – we are waiting praise the Lord!

But, while I wait, my heart is heavy. Tonight, Kathy and Alice told us about a crowd coming this morning to 'dechouké' (kill) Pastor Cebien because he had sent one of the orphans away. This orphan is over 20 years old and over six feet tall, and is not a child anymore. Pastor Cebien stood and argued amid their screams and yells for three hours. Alice was really impressed – she says the Lord has really been using him lately. Actually, the crowd was blaming Pastor Néonce and his wife for everything. They say that they have put 'magic' on Pastor Cebien and Kathy and Alice, so they can't see how bad the Néonces are.

Someone (they think another pastor) stole some of Pastor Cebien's benches, his generator, his accordion, and one of his pasta machines (they use them to make money selling pasta) from Champin the other night. Poor man, he tries so hard to build something, and then things like this happen. They also stole some cement. He is never discouraged, at least if he is, you would never see it or hear it from him.

June 1, 1989

So much has happened! All of our plans are set, tickets are bought, and I'll soon be leaving Haiti. My heart is ambivalent – I'm both sad and glad. Sad to be leaving people I love here, the excitement, the children, this house, the dog, the cat, and sad not being able to see my son Tom, while he is in the Dominican Republic. He just didn't let me know soon enough, I leave on the thirteenth, and he arrives on the fifteenth. Dr. Bibiana will arrive back here on the plane that I will leave on, so I will miss her too. These things all make me very sad.

Babiole was closed by the Health Department (I didn't even know there was one) two weeks ago, and now the kids are all coming to Morne Rouge. Kathy and Alice said, "See, if you'd closed Babiole before, you'd have a good clinic now!

Maybe they are right, but I really felt at the time that I had to keep it open. Maybe I made a mistake. I've probably made many! I just pray I'm not making one now.

These things have all just happened now. If they had happened a month ago, I probably would have stayed, but – they didn't, and I have to believe the Lord is still in control of all things. He knows what He is doing, even when we don't.

I had planned to go out on MFI on June twentieth but that date was filled, and so was the twenty-seventh. Skip had already bought tickets that couldn't be changed, so I will have to leave on the thirteenth.

I've had some good quality time talking with Pastor Cebien, and I know the Lord is speaking to him. He even prayed with me. I will miss him, and Kathy and Alice very, very much. We had our Bible study here tonight, and I will miss all of these folks as well.

Last Sunday, May twenty-eighth, was Mother's Day here in Haiti. It's a very big holiday, and everyone tries to have a new outfit to wear to church, rather like our Easter used to be. I went alone to Champin to hear Pastor Cebien preach. Appropriately, he preached on Mothers.

During his sermon, I could hear some chicken noises from the back door, and after a few minutes, a hen with two babies came into view. They seemed to like it there, and while he preached about Mothers, this little mother settled down and took her two babies under her wings in a perfect living illustration of the sermon. I don't know if anyone else in the congregation saw the illustration, but I thoroughly enjoyed it, and said, "Thank You Lord!"

June 12, 1989

I can't believe it's my last day in Haiti – Maybe forever. This last two weeks have been difficult in so many ways. There are so many people I will miss SO much, but there are so many things I will be glad to miss. The electricity is off again – that I won't miss. I saw a poor little horse down under his load – just lying there, probably dying. The poor animals here, seeing them suffering so – I won't miss! But the people, I will miss so much. They have become a part of my life I will never forget, and I just praise and thank the Lord for allowing me to have this time to learn a little better what the word – agape – means in everyday living. Self-sacrificing service to others. Last night I sang a duet with Pastor Cebien at church. Only for him would I sing – and then, it was really for the Lord.

I have everything packed – only last minute things left, and then, Lord willing – I'm gone.

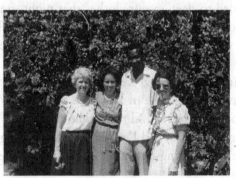

Left to right, me, Kathy, Pastor Cebien, and Alice

What Happened Next?

Yes, Skip and I were married in June of 1989. We lived near Rochester, New York, in the small town of Marion.

In 1990, Skip and I went back to Haiti to visit our friends there, and to look at the possibility of coming back to serve there together. It was not the Lord's will for us to do that, but while we were there, we got in on another coup.

The airport was closed, and there were several incidents in town with some of the merchants whose stores were trashed, and everything thrown out into the streets. One of those merchants lived in the house just in front of Flo's where we were staying. When it all started, he got in his car and drove home, but he parked his car out behind our house. My thought was, *"Great! When they come for him, they'll think he lives here, and we'll all get it."*

We all decided to sleep in our clothes that night so if they came, we could go out the back door and run up the mountain behind us, and get away. However, they didn't come, so all we lost was a night's sleep. Thanks to the Lord!

Since the airport was closed we couldn't get out, but MFI asked the airport for permission to come in and take out those who were told by their mission boards to leave, and those who wanted to leave. They were given permission to do this, and I've never seen anything as sweet as that old DC-3 as it came floating down out of the blue to the runway to take us home.

In 1991 Skip retired from Kodak, and we moved to Flagstaff, Arizona, where we joined The Navajo Gospel Mission. Skip was active in building and repairing the mission's churches, while giving the young men the benefit his years of expertise in 'how to do' plumbing, wiring, and many other facets of construction; at the same time he was teaching them the Scripture.

I was disappointed that I was unable to work as a nurse on the reservation due to government regulations, so I went to work at the local hospital, in the Newborn Nursery, and the Newborn Intensive Care Unit.

I took care of lots of new little Navajo babies. We worked and worshipped with many of the local missionaries, and fully enjoyed our life there.

Three years after we moved to Flagstaff, Skip had a mild heart attack. He suffered another major attack six months later, when he had gone for a walk in the woods alone, and this time, the Lord took him home.

My mother was now eighty-nine years old and living alone in Lake Montezuma, Arizona, about an hours drive away from Flagstaff. About a year after Skip had died, she began to have some medical problems, so we decided it was time for us to move in together so I could take care of her.

We bought a house in Big Pine, California, where we lived until my mother went to be with the Lord in 2005, when she was 97 years old.

After her death, I lived in our house for another year, and then I moved to Tonopah, Nevada; which is an oasis of an old gold and silver mining town, in the high desert, four hours north of Las Vegas, and four hours south of Reno. Our closest city of any size is Bishop, California, which is a two hour drive over the White Mountains.

I have two sons, two grand-children, and five great grand-children all living here, and I will probably still be here when the Lord calls me home to be with HIM.

Pastor Cebien, and Kathy and Alice are still faithfully serving in Morne Rouge at E.B.A.C. They felt the January earthquake, but there was very little damage in the north of Haiti, so they were spared that, though about a month later they were faced with the thousands of refugees moving north, and they were able to help with feeding them.

Flo had to leave when she was diagnosed with breast cancer, and has since died.

I have no idea of what has happened to Ronnie or any of the others that I worked with.

Oh, Yes. Remember the barrel that Skip put up on our roof? He put it up there so we would have water to shower when there was no electricity, and it worked wonderfully for a long time, and was much appreciated. Well, after I had been home for several months, I got a letter from Flo, asking me if maybe I would like to send them some money to help repair the roof.

Then she went on to say that the barrel had come through the roof and dumped thirty gallons of water on the floor in the house. She and Ma'Louie had spent about five hours mopping it up, and she was a bit unhappy with me. I felt pretty bad about it, and gladly sent her some money to help repair the roof. Well, it was a good idea, but the platform the barrel was sitting on shifted, and now you know the rest of the story.

If anyone has any questions about any thing I have written, please feel free to write to me, and I will try to answer them to the best of my remembrance, and thank you for reading my book. May God bless you and keep you!

My address to write to is:

Pat Bramhall

P.O. Box 1088, Tonopah, NV 89049-1088

haitipat@frontiernet.net